Intermittent Autophagy For Detox Your Body, Burn Fat Rapidly, Promote Longevity & Improve Hormonal Health For Men & Women + 5 Extreme Weight Loss Hypnosis

© **Copyright 2021 - All rights reserved.**

The content contained within this book may not be reproduced, duplicated or transmitted without direct written permission from the author or the publisher. Under no circumstances will any blame or legal responsibility be held against the publisher, or author, for any damages, reparation, or monetary loss due to the information contained within this book; either directly or indirectly.

Legal Notice:

This book is copyright protected. This book is only for personal use. You cannot amend, distribute, sell, use, quote or paraphrase any part, or the content within this book, without the consent of the author or publisher.

Disclaimer Notice:

Please note the information contained within this document is for educational and entertainment purposes only. All effort has been executed to present accurate, up to date, and reliable, complete information. No warranties of any kind are declared or implied. Readers acknowledge that the author is not engaging in the rendering of legal, financial, medical or professional advice.

TABLE OF CONTENTS

INTRODUCTION **5**

SECTION 1: AUTOPHAGY AND FASTING **14**

   CHAPTER ONE: Autophagy 15

   CHAPTER TWO: Fasting 27

   CHAPTER THREE: Breaking a Fast 51

   CHAPTER FOUR: Fats and Cholesterol 70

SECTION 2: HORMONES AND HORMONAL IMBALANCE **83**

   CHAPTER FIVE: Hormones 84

   CHAPTER SIX: Hormonal Imbalance 93

   CHAPTER SEVEN: Hormones and Heredity 108

SECTION 3: DETOXING **120**

   CHAPTER EIGHT: Cleanses and Other Detox Programs 121

   CHAPTER NINE: Popular Cleanses 149

SECTION 4: DIETING **160**

   CHAPTER TEN: Ketogenic Diet 161

CHAPTER ELEVEN: Other Popular Diets 178

CHAPTER TWELVE: Natural Supplements 218

SECTION 5: EXERCISE 228

CHAPTER THIRTEEN: Exercising During Fasts 229

SECTION 6: YOGA FOR FASTING 257

CHAPTER FOURTEEN: Yoga for Fasting 258

CHAPTER FIFTEEN: A Program for Yoga During Fasting 269

SECTION 7: MEDITATION FOR FASTING 306

CHAPTER SIXTEEN: Meditation for Fasting 307

CHAPTER SEVENTEEN: Meditation Programs for Fasting and the Immunity System 331

SECTION 8: HYPNOTISM 341

CHAPTER EIGHTEEN: Hypno-fasting 342

CHAPTER NINETEEN: Hypnosis Programs 355

CONCLUSION 434

RESOURCES 441

INTRODUCTION

The World Health Organization estimates that 700 million adults are obese. It's linked to roughly five million deaths around the world yearly, roughly eight percent of global deaths per year. Thirteen percent of adults worldwide are obese and thirty-nine percent are overweight. One in five children and adolescents are overweight all over the world.

Experts estimate that over 34 million people (over ten percent of the population of the United States, have diabetes. Roughly 26.8 million people (also over ten percent of the population) had diagnosed diabetes and over seven million people have the disease but have not been diagnosed.

Hormonal imbalances strike both men and women (women at a whopping 80%).

There's no doubt that our fast-paced, nutrient-deficient world has wrought havoc on our bodies. Pollutants corrupt and weaken our immune systems, our cells cannot engage in the necessary process of autophagy, which recycles usable cellular materials and discards toxins and unusable cellular waste. This affects everything else in the body and in the mind, creating downward spirals which can take your entire future with it, swirling down the drain like a tubful of dirty water.

On the other hand, there are ways to combat and even reverse the corrosive effects of having a toxified body and mind. It's widely known in the medical field that people who engage in regular physical exercise have:

A 30% lower risk of early death

- Roughly 50% lowered risk of type 2 diabetes
- Roughly 35% lowered risk of stroke and coronary disease
- Roughly 50% lowered risk of colon cancer
- Roughly 20% lowered risk of breast cancer

Fasting is also a powerful weapon for weight loss and overall good health. A review study illustrated that people who participated in intermittent fasting cut between four and seven percent from their waist measurements over a period of six months.

So there little doubt that there are a number of natural remedies for these life-threatening conditions. This book is your guide to these and other remedies for these and other conditions! This book will give you the history, the latest information and the results of the most cutting-edge studies and experiments. You'll learn everything you need to know (and you do need to know it) about autophagy, fasting and hormonal imbalances. You'll put into practice the leading methods of weight loss and general good health; cleansing and detox, dieting, exercise, yoga, meditation, and even hypnotism. You will obtain a working knowledge of good health from the molecular level all the way to full-body longevity. You'll learn what to eat and what not to eat, and why! You'll learn how your body works, how your mind works, and how they work together. But you'll do more than learn, you'll *do*, putting these concepts into real action which will change your body, your mind, your entire life.

These exercises come from the leading experts in their field, the programs chosen specifically to address the maladies this book is written to address. So you don't have to sift through information which may be valuable but not precisely relevant. The data comes from the world's most trusted sources (The World Health Organization, for one). This book, like all our books, is held to the highest standard of excellence and integrity, making complex medical information easy to understand and making complex concepts easy to ingest. We've helped countless readers improve their lives, shedding light on everything from true leadership skills to various mental disorders and much, much more. Readers come to us time and again to help them remedy the things which plague their lives, the things which plague so many lives. This book addresses the discrepancy between body and soul, between temporary satisfaction and true happiness.

But the benefits are a lot more specific than that. Sure, we can promise you long-lasting good health and mental stability, but the question of how to achieve them will also be answered. It's not just about what, but how, and this book will walk you, step-by-step, through processes you'll come across. Wellness is the destination at the end of your journey, and we'll take that journey with you and be with you every step of the way.

The statistics prove that these approaches work. Generations of longevity demonstrate the fact. New technology now illuminates what was once misunderstood or even unknown to modern science. But these things have finally caught up with the advancing technologies which create processed foods, electronic light, a barrage of media, Now you'll have a fighting chance against industrial superpowers who make fortunes from shortening the lives of people like you and me.

In fact, there's so much diverse information here, just one lesson well-learned could change your entire life. If you read and understand the chapter on fats and cholesterol alone, you'll have learned the difference between good cholesterol and bad (a difference which even now may be taking you by surprise). That alone could make the difference between your life and your death. Even understanding what autophagy is and how it works is worth the price of entry, as it will change the way you look at your body and your life. It's your body, shouldn't you know how it works? It's your mind, shouldn't you know how to use it?

Instinctively, you know these things to be true. It's why you're reading this introduction and deciding whether or not to buy and read this book. But even deeper down, you realize you haven't got a choice. If you're looking for a remedy, that means the problem has been going on for some time now. Even as you read this, your blood may be thickening while your bones become hollow and brittle. You're eating things you want but don't need, and every heartbeat could be your last. You may be living on the precipice of a heart attack or stroke. Or you may simply be looking at the slow decline which will rob you of the idealized life you've worked so hard for. Don't let that dream die, don't let your body die. Your health is in your hands, both figuratively and literally. If you don't do it now, when will you? It's easy to procrastinate, to think nothing will work (we have a book about that too). But it's vital that you take the crucial next step. You've already taken the first step, and that's to seek help. The next step is to accept that help, and the other steps are delineated in this book. Follow them, but don't follow them blindly. As we point out in this book, this is a guide. But you'll still want to follow your doctor's recommendations, do other research. Questions will arise, and no book can anticipate every question you may have. So take the hunger to learn which this book will help you develop and let that carry over to other research, other forms of due diligence. It's your overall wellbeing, and you are responsible for it. But again, you won't have to do it alone. We're here for you as long as you are there for yourself.

And it's not just about you. Because chances are that, even if you are in constant control and perfect health, you know somebody who isn't. The statistics bare this out. So if you're concerned about someone else, the information in this book is even more vital. You may already be convinced that there's a problem. But all too often those who have these problems are in denial. This book is designed to turn them around, to change their outlooks and set them on the journey toward a better and longer and healthier life.

But will they do as they're told? Not likely. You have to lead by example. So consider adopting some of these practices even if your weight and muscular integrity are in fine shape. You can always do better. Stress always comes up in life, and that can cause inflammation and related diseases. Good health is a matter of mindfulness and deliberate action. We can all always be more mindful, more deliberate, and be in even better mental or physical health, no matter where we are on the spectrum of good health. All we need is information, inspiration, and dedication.

So just do it. Don't waste another second. Read this book, do these exercises, engage in these practices, Share it with your friends. They'll all want to know what you're doing once you turn up leaner and happier and healthier, with clear skin and a vibrant glow. They'll beg to know your secrets, and you'll be well-prepared to share them. You're about to lead them down a road to wellness you or they may never have known existed. But now you hold the roadmap. Look down; your feet already taking the first few steps. Now you take the rest; we'll take them together.

Now let's get started!

SECTION 1: AUTOPHAGY AND FASTING

CHAPTER ONE: Autophagy

Autophagy is the human body's method of flushing out damaged cells, so as to regenerate new, healthy cells. It's easier to remember than you may think; *auto* refers to *self*, such as in *automatic*, and *phagy,* meaning *to eat*. Some people even think of autophagy as *self-devouring,* and we'll soon see why that's actually highly beneficial and even essential to good health.

Not only does autophagy remove dysfunctional cells, it can recycle some parts of those cells and use them for cellular cleaning and repair by use of organelles called *autophagosomes*. This process binds unwanted cellular matter with other cellular components called lysosomes. A lysosome releases acidic enzymes which break the material down, allowing some materials to be reused while others are discarded.

Autophagy Genes

The pathway of lysosomal autophagy degradation clearly plays a huge role in organismal, tissue, and cellular homeostasis. It's mediated by certain genes called autophagy-related (ATG) genes. There are definitive etiological links between mutations in the genes which control autophagy and also human disease, particularly cancer, and certain genomic, cardiovascular, neurodegenerative and inflammatory disorders. Autophagy targets dysfunctional organelles, pathogenic proteins, and intracellular microbes. ATG genes have many roles of considerable physiological importance. It also plays vital roles in other membrane trafficking and in signaling critical lysosomal pathways.

There are actually least three distinct types of autophagy, including chaperone-mediated, microautophagy, and macroautophagy. They differ as the mode of delivery of the rejected cargo to the lysosome. Macroautophagy is the primary mechanism which is used by eukaryotic cells in order to maintain nutrient homeostasis and organellar quality control.

Benefits of Autophagy

Autophagy was only discovered as recently as the 1960s, in human liver cells, and has been associated with a variety of other organs and tissues as well.

One of the first and most evident benefits of autophagy manifest in what seem to be anti-aging effects. This is so because autophagy helps replace old cells with new ones, maintaining the body's youthful functioning and appearance.

Autophagy also removes toxic cellular proteins which are associated with Alzheimer's and Parkinson's diseases and other neurodegenerative diseases.

Autophagy also recycles these residual proteins to provide energy and other options for cellular repair, as well as prompting the regeneration of healthy cells.

Autophagy is on the frontline of cancer research and treatment. This only makes perfect sense, as cancer is basically the uncontrolled reproduction of dysfunctional cells, and autophagy is the process of flushing out and recycling damaged cells to prevent their proliferation. Autophagy seems to slow down as we age; likewise, the likelihood of cancer increases as we age. The connection between autophagy and cancer is theoretical at the moment, with little hard evidence to back it up.

In fact, a study in 2019 found that autophagy can stall cancer cell development, it may promote their growth as well. This appears contingent on the stage of the tumor.

A 2020 review article suggests that autophagy may help protect liver cells from alcohol- and drug-induced injury to the liver. It may also prevent or limit the progression of several dangerous liver conditions, such as Wilson's disease, nonalcoholic fatty liver, chronic alcohol abuse-related liver disease.

Autophagy may also play a vital role in the human immune system as it cleans out infectious agents and toxins. It may also control inflammation, which may help manage cells with neurodegenerative or infectious diseases and protect them from incoming microbes.

When cells are stressed, autophagy increases, allowing the body to survive and even to thrive. Starvation is just one of these stresses, and it apparently encourages autophagy, according to experts. And this only makes sense; when the body has nothing else to eat, it eats itself. This is how stores of body fat are burned for useful energy. Cells are recycled and reused when necessary, and in basically the same way. It's not a sustainable survival method, but it can be life-saving in times of crisis.

Diet and Autophagy

Autophagy is unquestionably related to diet. And it's not just about what you eat and when, but if you eat at all.

And better diet and weight control are more necessary now than ever. Obesity affected 13% of adults globally in 2016.

Obesity is often the catalyst of metabolic syndrome which is a cluster of metabolic abnormalities. These include high blood pressure, type 2 diabetes, high blood pressure, and low HDL (good) cholesterol. We've already seen the terrifying statistics on global obesity.

So weight management and loss are important to good health, and autophagy is crucial to weight management and loss. That brings us to the dietary specifics of autophagy.

The first dietary change associated with autophagy is intermittent fasting. Having nothing else to eat, the body will recycle stored fats, proteins, and cellular nutrients. Again, this isn't a sustainable way of survival, but it does kickstart the process of autophagy. We'll take a closer look at fasting in a moment.

Ketosis, or the keto diet, is a diet often associated with autophagy. Because it restricts caloric intake of carbohydrates, it stimulates the body's use of reserves to burn energy. In the keto diet, roughly 75% of the body's calories come from fat and only five to ten percent from carbohydrates. This shift causes the body to change certain metabolic pathways. The body then begins to use fat for fuel rather than the glucose which is derived from carbohydrates. This shift in metabolism is what is known as ketosis.

Given the limitation of carbs, the body produces ketone bodies which provide a variety of benefits, such as breaking up fats.

The keto diet and intermittent fasting are both associated with low glucose levels, low insulin levels, and high glucagon levels. It's the glucagon level which is of interest here, as this initiates autophagy. Low sugar levels cause the kind of positive stress which triggers autophagy.

Exercise also plays a key role in triggering autophagy. And this only makes good sense. Exercise burns calories and causes the body to devour its resources, especially given a restriction of new carbohydrates. Autography from physical exercise is prevalent in organs which play a part in the metabolic processes, such as the pancreas, liver, muscles, and adipose tissue (body fat).

Curcumin, found in the turmeric root, is a popular spice in foods around the world and is often found in East Indian foods. Curcumin is associated with good health and long life.

A study using animals found a link between autophagy with a heavy reliance on curcumin may prevent diabetic cardiomyopathy, which is a heart muscle disorder affecting sufferers of diabetes. A different study using mice suggests that curcumin was useful in helping fight the cognitive impairment resultant from chemotherapy. It does this by inducing autophagy in specific brain regions.

But scientists stop short of asserting that increasing one's curcumin intake has a direct connection to inducing autophagy in the human body.

Studies have also shown that insulin, unsurprisingly, prevents autophagy. Insulin is released in response to food intake, and since fasting induces autophagy, eating and insulin release would be expected to hinder it. IGF-1 (or insulin-like growth factor) which increases with overall protein intake, also seems to inhibit autophagy.

A moderate amount of coffee is associated with the reduced risk of several diseases and chronic conditions. It may help prevent type 2 diabetes, protect against dementia. It carries essential nutrients like:

- Pantothenic acid (vitamin B5), providing 6% reference daily intake (RDI)
- Riboflavin (vitamin B2), providing 11% RDI
- Magnesium and niacin (vitamin B3), providing 2% RDI
- Manganese and potassium, providing 3% RDI

Coffee has an unusual effect on autophagy. In a study done on mice, coffee increased restorative activity during fasting. On the one hand, fasting invokes repair and rest. But coffee activates the liver.

Many experts agree that coffee should not be ingested during a water fast.

It's important to note here that any major change in diet should be preceded by a consultation with a physician. Pregnancy, heart conditions, diabetes, or hereditary traits should all be taken in to consideration before any significant change in a diet or exercise regiment.

Side Effects and Risks of Autophagy

We've taken a look at the benefits of autophagy. But even that has brushed us up against some of the unknown qualities and quantities of the process, including the promotion of cancerous tumor cells. So let's take a closer look at the other risks and possible side effects of autophagy.

The first thing it's important to note is the difference between the risks associated with the actual process of autophagy on one hand, and the risks involved with an individual's efforts to induce the process of autophagy.

First, the risks of autophagy itself are considerable. Studies have shown that autophagy in excess may damage heart cells. Links have been established between various heart problems and excessive autophagy.

As we looked at briefly, autophagy and cancer are closely associated. And while there may be anti-cancer benefits to limited autophagy, studies using mice showed that inhibiting autophagy limited tumor growth. This suggests that autophagy may contribute to tumor growth.

Fasting and Autophagy

How long should a person fast to achieve the so-called *autophagic flux*, the shift occurring in autophagy? Experts suggest between three and five days but not longer.

Studies done on mice show that fasting can result in autophagy in various organs, including the heart, the liver, and the brain. Mice who fasted for 24 hours showed neuronal autophagy, and it only increased after a total of 48 hours. Another study with mice showed that 18 of fasting resulted in autophagic structures in liver cells.

One human study demonstrated a 30% increase in LC3-II, an autophagic marker, after 72 hours of fasting. It also increased p62, another autophagy marker of autophagy, p62. A different study demonstrated that human volunteers who fasted for four days had increases in autophagic activity the most abundant human white blood cells, called *neutrophils*. But other types of white blood cells did not show similarly increased activity.

That's a good rundown of autophagy. It's important to know because it's at the heart of everything we're going to look at from this point forward. It is at the very center of what we're doing it, how we're doing it, and why. It's the body's natural mechanism of renewal. It's the cornerstone of what we're building, a tower of good mental and physical health. But for now, let's take an even closer look at fasting, long-term and short-term, the benefits and the drawbacks.

CHAPTER TWO: Fasting

Fasting is an ancient practice of self-denial. It's often spiritual and sometimes political, but for our purposes it's mostly dietary. That doesn't mean the psychological aspect isn't important, in fact its crucial. Fasting is where body and mind will meet, as we'll see soon enough. But for now lets look at the particular parts and then pull back to see how they all work together. First up was autophagy. We now know how important it is to good health. Fasting is one of the very best ways of instigating autophagy, which puts it next on our list.

Some of the benefits of fasting include:

- Gut health
- Heart health
- Brain health
- Body composition
- Energy levels
- Immune system health
- Appetite regulation

- Anti-aging and longevity
- Willpower, self-control, and relationship with food

There are different types of fasts for different results, and these depend largely on the maladies a person might be suffering, from obesity to toxicity. Different fasts can have different results.

If your goal is general digestive health: caloric liquid fasting (CLF) is best. This intermediate-level practice requires the faster to consume low-calorie liquids only (bone broth, low-sugar juices, water, unsweetened coffee and tea). These fasts may last been one and five days and may have potent effects on the strength of digestion and flora in the gut.

If you're fasting for longevity, a non-caloric liquid fast is an advanced fast which allows only non-caloric beverages (unsweetened coffee, tea, and water). One can go on with a fast like this for between one and seven days, but no more. The cellular cleanse of this approach is ideal for autophagy. We'll talk more about these in a moment.

For body composition, intermittent fasting is probably best. Which we'll now discuss in far greater detail.

We basically break up fasting into two cycles; intermittent or short-term fasting, and long-term fasting, and there are a few variations on both of those. Our focus in this book is intermittent fasting, so we'll take a look at that first.

Note: Whatever fast you choose, precede a fast with a period of light eating. Let the transition period be half of the anticipated fasting period. If you're planning a one-day fast, eat light the half-day before. Preceded a week-long fast with three-and-a-half days of light eating. The body will be prepared for the drop-off, which will not seem as steep and hard to manage.

Intermittent Fasting

We've already seen some of the benefits of autophagy, and they're closely related to the same benefits of intermittent fasting. They include weight loss (belly fat), improved organ health, muscle strength, improved metabolism, and overall longevity.

A 2014 review study showed that intermittent fasting may generate three to eight percent weight loss over three to 24 weeks. Similar studies show the same thing, but to lesser degrees. Intermittent fasting is known to boost norepinephrine, which elevates the metabolic rate, from roughly four percent to roughly 14%.

Intermittent fasting is also known to increase Human Growth Hormone (HGH). This hormone (and we'll take a closer look at them later) helps prevent muscle loss which happens during weight loss. It also boosts insulin levels, increasing availability of body fat as fuel. This is key to ketosis, the center of the ketogenic diet, which we'll also look at in greater detail. It's one of the premiere diets for before and after fasts and cleansing.

Intermittent Fasting and Weight Loss

Intermittent fasting has a demonstrable effect on weight loss, as we've seen. And while intermittent fasting has many other benefits to the human body, weight loss is certainly one of them.

Before we go much further, it's important to note that fasting of any sort is not recommended for women who are pregnant, anyone under the age of 18, sufferers of diabetes or low blood pressure, or who may have an eating disorder or a history of the same.

Losing weight is basically about burning more calories than you consume. To do this, one generally changes their diet to reduce caloric intake while changing their exercise regiment to burn more calories. There's no particular mystery to that.

But the body isn't that simple, as we've seen with just a cursory look at autophagy, and as we'll see in much greater detail later in this book. For now, let's agree that there's a bit more to losing weight than caloric balance. There's also more to intermittent fasting than just losing weight. We've already taken a brief look at how intermittent fasting triggers autophagy, keeping organs healthy and encouraging longevity.

But there is still the matter of weight loss and intermittent fasting.

First of all, it's important to understand what factors may affect weight loss. They include:

- Sleep
- Age
- Gender
- Stress
- Genetics
- Medication
- Hormones
- Microbiome
- Metabolic rate
- Health status
- Food quality

These things affect satiety, appetite, and energy levels, which determine calorie intake and processing.

Intermittent fasting (sometimes called time-restricted feeding), is more an eating schedule than a classic diet. It's less about *what* you eat, but *when* you eat … and when you *don't*.

As an example, the 16/8 intermittent fast requires 16 hours of fasting followed by an eight-hour eating window. period during which you consume all of your daily calories. Other popular variations include 13/11, 18/16, and 20/4. We'll take a closer look at these and other shortly.

It's important to note that, while intermittent fasting is a powerful weight-loss tool, there are no studies which show that it is more effective than other weight-loss regiments. We'll take a look at other potent and popular diet regiments later in this book.

For now, let's keep our focus on intermittent fasting and its effects on weight loss. Some of the benefits of intermittent fasting for weight loss include:

- Easy: As you'll see, it's easier to follow than counting calories

- Flexible: Different methods of intermittent fasting (IF) can be made to fit any lifestyle
- Self-awareness: Learning the difference between physiological and psychological hunger
- Self-control: Limiting eating windows requires and encourages discipline

What about the drawbacks of intermittent fasting? Not everybody loses weight with intermittent fasting. Why is that?

Premenopausal women may or may not lose weight with intermittent fasting, and it can even be detrimental to some. It's for this reason we don't recommend it for premenopausal women. We have another book like this one, focusing on fasting for women, and it has more in-depth information.

Overeating during the eating windows is another reason some people fail to lose weight. It's important not to eat too much, and to eat food which is as healthy as possible. Limiting alcohol intake is also crucial to weight loss with intermittent fasting and is recommended for organ health.

Insufficient exercise may limit weight loss during an intermittent fast. While we'll explain later how vigorous exercise can be detrimental to the body during fasts. But some exercise (walking, for example) can be beneficial and will prevent muscle atrophy.

Different Methods of Intermittent Fasting

There are several popular ways of short-term fasting. One popular way to do is known as *the 16/8 method.* Also known as *the Leangains protocol,* this method is simple to follow: Daily fasting for between 14 and 16 hours with an 8- to 10-hour eating window. The eating window may allow for two or more meals of healthy foods low in carbohydrates.

It may sound like a lot of math (or maths, if you like) but it's really not far from the average dietary cycle. For example, if your eating window opens at 8 am, it closes at 6 pm. That's really just a matter of eating an early dinner and cutting out the midnight snacks. For some reason, women seem to do better with a shorter fasting block and longer eating window, of between 14 and 15 hours.

Water, coffee, and drinks with zero-calories can be consumed during the fasting blocks.

Variations on this approach include 13/11 (13 hours fasting with an 11-hour eating window), 18/16 (18 hours fasting with a 16-hour eating window) and 20/4 (20 hours fasting with a four-hour eating window).

These seem increasingly complex, and they can be harder to follow that the first approach. In point of fact, they're really not. Look at them this way: The 13-hour fasting approach may begin at noon and end at one in the morning. That offers an 11-hour eating window which lasts until noon the next day. It's basically a breakfast-and-early-lunch cycle, that's not so hard to follow. The 20/4 approach give the faster a regular eating window for whatever their preferred meal; a long breakfast, lunch, or dinner period. Work schedules may make the dinner hours the best for the 20/4 approach. The 18/16 approach is tricker because it's not a straight 24-hour cycle. This approach staggers the schedule, so you're basically having breakfast one day, lunch the next day, dinner the next day. Once the faster falls into that regular schedule, it's still easier to remember than more complex diet plans, which we'll look at later in this book.

Another method of short-term fasting is *the 5/2 diet*. This method divides the week into two blocks of five days and two days. Dieters eat they normally would, but then severely restrict their caloric intake for the other two days.

Keep in mind that the two days do not have to be sequential, though they may be. A dieter may choose to separate them, often on Mondays and Thursdays, for example. Many dieters appreciate the weekends as times to celebrate and eat normally and find weekdays better days to sacrifice comfort foods. Those two days might include two small meals of 250-300 calories each (men are recommended to intake just a bit more calories than women).

There is also the *Eat Stop Eat* method. This is basically the habit of fasting for 24 hours on a periodic basis. Dieters may eat at 6 pm on one day, then fast until dinner the next night. It's little more than skipping breakfast and lunch for one day, maybe once or twice week. If a dieter prefers breakfast, they can eat a big breakfast and then fast until the next morning and eat a reasonable breakfast along with other meals latter that day. Water and coffee and zero-calorie beverages are allowed during fasting times, but naturally no solid food.

Eating regularly during non-fasting days is important. Don't double-up on regular days to make up for fasting. The whole idea is to limit caloric intake and encourage the body to draw on its resources, not add to the stored energy.

Note that 24 hours can be a long time for a lot of novice dieters. Newbies might try a 16-hour fast at first and then expand that block as they become more comfortable.

Alternate-day fasting is just what it sounds; one day of regular eating followed by one day of fasting (or very limited intake, 500-600 calories max). As a lot of people prefer a week-long cycle, a lot of alternate-day fasters both start and end the week on regular eating days, comprising a total of four regular days and three fasting days in the week, with Sunday and Monday being two regular eating days in a row.

This can be a punishing regiment for beginners and is recommended for advanced dieters.

The Warrior Diet made popular by fitness guru Ori Hofmekler, finds the dieter eating small portions of raw vegetables and fruits throughout the day and then one big meal at night. This allows for a four-hour eating window at the end of the day, preferably not too late. This is one of the most popular types of intermittent fasting.

Spontaneous meal-skipping is one of the most forgiving types of intermittent fasting. It involves the dieter occasionally skipping meals. It's a myth that the human being needs to eat every couple of hours. So the dieter skips a meal irregularly. Let your daily schedule dictate what to skip. Interruptions and crises will arise, so take care of them and let that midday meal slide past. It won't kill you … in fact, it just might save your life.

The health risks and drawbacks to short-term fasting seem limited, temporary, and manageable. They may include dizziness or lightheadedness, distractedness, inability to concentrate, and nausea.

Long-term Fasting

While short-term fasting often includes a full day without eating (but not without drinking some beverages), long-term fasting may go on for two days or more.

A *dry fast* is the most extreme type of long-term fasting, wherein the dieter consumes no food or beverage of any kind, including water. We don't recommend this, as it can have terrible effects on the body, including liver and kidney damage, skin damage, tooth loss, and heart problems. Twenty-four hours is as long as anyone should go without drinking something.

Water fasting is like dry fasting but with water. No calories are ingested in this type of long-term fasting. Water fasting means drinking only water, but consuming no calories during the fast.

A comparable technique is juice fasting wherein only fruit or vegetable juices are consumed. A variation on this technique is the broth fast, which provides liquid and minimal caloric intake. But neither juice fasting nor broth fasting are true fasting. Keep in mind that intermittent fasting isn't strictly fasting either if you're drinking coffee during your fasting periods.

But protein has to be accompanied by some fat to help break it down for our human digestive systems. Native Americans used to cook and eat rabbits whole, eating the eyes, the brains, any source of fat the animal could offer.

Let's turn our attention to water fasting, which is common and effective in a lot of ways.

Weight loss is among the most prominent effects of water fasting. One day of fasting uses the liver's storage of glycogen, and the body turns to reserves after that; either fat or protein.

Fasters may lose one to two pounds per day of water weight. Proteins are used by the body first, but this can mean a breakdown in muscles before the fat reserved is tapped. Fat is the preferred fuel for this reason. Once the excess proteins are used, the body draws on fat reserves and converts that to energy. Fat is more energy-dense than protein, so weight loss slows as the fat is being burned off, at a rate of roughly one pound every two days.

While long-term fasting is a powerful tool for weight loss, it's important to note that the weight often returns after the fast. This happens because the dieter often returns to bad eating habits, too many carbs and sugars to create glutenous fat. So once the body is in a state of ketosis, looking to fat as a fuel, it's important to keep it up and not revert to old ways of eating.

A study of obese patients who reported weight loss during two weeks' fasting found that half of the patients either failed to return a follow-up call, indicating that they'd put the weight back on, or that they'd put the weight back on within two years.

Long-term fasts have other benefits too. Like intermittent fasting, long-term fasting promotes autophagy, which we already know has multiple health benefits.

One study found benefits to sufferers of hypertension of extended fasts (an average of ten days) and of cancer patients undergoing chemotherapy (an average of five days).

Long-term fasting may also allow a dieter to reset their relationship with their favorite foods. Once physically away from the comforting crutches of sugar snacks and massive meals, the dieter my find that they find solace in other, healthier ways.

The dangers and risks of long-term fasting are more drastic than those related to short-term fasting. One of the most considerable risks of long-term fasting, it should surprise nobody, is starving to death. It's unusual unless deliberate, as in a hunger strike, which can last between 46 and 73 days.

Short of that, there still serious risks. Fasting stresses the heart by cannibalizing cardiac muscles for fuel. Muscle is the first sacrifice of fasting until the body shifts to ketosis. Heart failure may occur in extreme cases, and long-term damage to the heart muscles becomes increasingly likely as long-term fasting continues.

But long-term fasting and heart damage has a second, and dangerous aspect. The body uses its store of potassium and magnesium. When combined with muscular compromise, these mineral deficiencies can be fatal.

Infectious diseases can also be a threat to long-term fasters, as they lack the nutrition for a strong immune system.

Less dangerous risks include low energy, mood swings, irritability, and an increase in cortisol and norepinephrine, stress hormones. This can cause a fasting high, encouraging more (and more dangerous) fasting.

Another drawback to long-term fasting is the rate the body detoxifies. Fat stores toxins, and fasting releases these toxins into the blood, causing nausea and sickness. The more rapid the detox, the more dangerous it can be.

One study followed a monk's 40-day fast, consuming roughly 60 calories per day from communion. After 36 days, the man had lost just short of 40 pounds, developed hypotension (low blood pressure). He had no significant changes in serum magnesium, potassium, phosphorous, or calcium, but did show a slight bump in serum zinc and uric acid, which stabilized in the third week and then normalized.

Intermittent fasting as certain advantages, including practicality, sociability, personal comfort. It forgoes the drawbacks of muscle loss, malnutrition, infectious diseases, and heart failure.

The long-term fast can have radical effects on the faster's perspective about food, ending lifelong cycles of malnutrition and bad diet, eating disorders, and food-related conditions like obesity and type-2 diabetes. It also leads the faster to confront the emotional causes of eating disorders.

Still-growing children should not fast; they need constant nutrition to healthy development. The elderly should also not fast, as they're likely to have inadequate stores of energy or may have advanced heart conditions which would put them at risk of heart failure. Sufferers of chronic problems with the heart or kidneys should not fast, nor should pregnant women or women trying to get pregnant.

If you're going to engage in a long-term fast, here are some tips:

- Talk to your doctor first about your goals and timeline.
- Explain to your friends and family to help socialize you so you don't have to be isolated.
- Get a fasting counselor or coach, or look into fasting groups.
- Integrate yoga and meditation.
- Integrate supplements of potassium, sodium, phosphate, calcium, and magnesium.
- Forgo vigorous exercise during fasting periods.

Fasting Apps

There are lots of fasting apps, and we don't have the time to run through them all. We're setting some which are designed specifically for women for our book on fasting for women, but there are plenty which are good for both men and women, and each has its benefits. All are free to download for Windows or IOs.

Zero is a popular app with a variety of valuable benefits:
- Easy customization of your fast
- Easy tracking of fasting progress and goals
- Easy journal entry for the completion of fasts
- Easy integrate with smart devices and wearables such as Apple Watch to monitor heart rate, weight, resting, and sleep

Fasting Tracker also has a number of handy benefits, including:
- Easy adjustment of fasting duration
- Easy logging of waist size, weight, ketones and glucose

- All access to in-app community for support
- Articles and videos

BodyFast offers some unique features, including:

- Fasting timer
- Fasting coach
- Weight tracker
- Statistics
- No advertisements
- Notification alerts
- Sharing progress
- Staying accountable to friends on various popular social platforms

Vora offers:

- Daily fast tracking
- Diet plan
- Tracking others' progress for inspiration
- Export data to CVS

Fastient offers:

- Ways to visualize fasting progress
- Ways to journal about your fasting progress and experience

- Ways to check fasting history
- Ways to import previous fasts from comparable apps
- Emojis
- Quick-tag
- Progress pictures
- Dark mode

FastHabit allows the users to:

- Stop, restart, or even to adjust fast
- Visualize progress in percentages
- Keep records of weight log
- Set fasting reminders and then get notified

Well, that was quite a bit of information, wasn't it? We've learned about autophagy, and the various ways of fasting in order to instigate and maintain it. You should have a greater working understanding of fasting than you had before, more than others around you have. Now you must start putting it to use. You may already have decided what kind of fasting is best for you, or you may not have made up your mind. Either way, that's great! Knowing what you want and need will help you to set the goal and achieve it. If you're not sure yet, it means you're on the journey to discovery. This book will give you all the information you need to make the right choice at the right time. And, as you'll see, it's a choice you can always adjust at any time, and go on adjusting as your understanding and as your needs change.

But whatever type of fasting you choose, you'll have to break that fast sometime, and that brings us to our next chapter; breaking a fast.

CHAPTER THREE:
Breaking a Fast

When you're ready to break your fast, you have to be careful. Too much food too soon can lead to refeeding syndrome. If your body undertakes the shift from ketosis to carbohydrate-based foods cause the body to release insulin for digestion, a process that requires phosphate, magnesium, calcium, potassium, and a variety of essential vitamins, particularly B1. Severe deficiencies can lead to heart failure and hypotension, sometimes leading to sudden death.

When refeeding, your body stimulates stem cell regeneration, as well as boosting hormones, immune system cells, and metabolic activity.

Here are some verified guidelines on avoiding refeeding syndrome when breaking a fast:

Start off by eating no more than ten calories per kilogram (daily) of body weight or less for breaking longer fasts.

Supplement with vitamins and minerals as described and take them a half-hour before breaking your fast.

Eat bone broth or pure fruit juice to break the fast. Follow up with pureed soups, avocados, well-cooked vegetables. Avoid fruits, as the fructose could be punishing on an empty stomach.

Eat smaller portions but more often, and eat slowly.

Those are the simplest guidelines. But fasting and then breaking that fast is about more than eating or not eating. It's about resetting your body, even on a molecular level. But it's also about resetting your relationship with food. As we've touched on (and will again), there is psychological eating and there is physiological eating, and the differences are plain.

Physiological eating is:
- Necessary
- Healthy
- Deliberate
- Motivated by physical need for food

While psychological eating is:

- Unnecessary
- Unhealthy
- Habitual
- Motivated by psychological need for comfort or distraction

So when breaking a fast, keep in mind that your relationship with food should fundamentally change from a psychological relationship to a physiological relationship.

In order to gain and secure over your eating habits and redefine your relationship with food, consider asking yourself these four questions:

His method involves asking yourself the following four questions:

1. Why? Why are you eating? If you're at the end of a feeding window and think of packing in a few extra mouthfuls simply because it's allowed, you may be eating for the wrong reason. Holidays, celebrations, and vacations are classic excuses to overeat, but that rarely makes any of those occasions more enjoyable and it certainly doesn't do anything

to maintain proper bodily metabolism or healthy autophagy.

Other bad reasons for eating include boredom, sadness, tiredness, and even thirst (often mistaken for hunger).

Consider alternatives to eating in these instances, including taking a walk or spending time with friends and family. Call them on the phone, there's an old-fashioned thought.

2. What? What are you eating? Because of the new stem cells being created after a fast, it's important to break a fast with the right foods. Some prefer organic foods, some may adhere to a food regiment like the ketogenic diet. But don't break your fast with junk food, no matter how much you think you may deserve it. In fact, you deserve better. Garbage in, garbage out; that's more important after a fast or cleanse than at any other time.

Remember your goals and let what you eat support those goals. If your goal was ketosis, don't load up on carbs. If weight loss is your goal, don't load up on fats unless you're on the ketogenic diet.

Be mindful and deliberate of what you eat, don't just fall into old habits.

3. How? How are you eating? As we pointed out briefly before, eating slowly is important. It gives your body to digest at its own pace and not be overwhelmed. Also, eating slowly is likely to create the feeling of being full without eating as great a quantity of food. This is more difficult and more important than ever in our fast-paced world of drive-thru convenience that delivers the most unhealthy foods right into our hands with limited time to consume them. The whole idea of a drive-thru is to eat on-the-go, but this is not how your body usually feeds and digests. The human body prefers a parasympathetic state. It would rather rest and digest in body and mind.

So be mindful of, well, your state of mind when you're eating, and the state of your body too. You might think of restricting your eating windows to the healthiest times, limiting late-night snacking. Eating in the morning, midday, or early evening is best. And when you are eating, try not to do other things. Avoid watching TV or working at a computer. These distractions interrupt mindful eating, and that's what this is all about. Know what you're eating, why, when, and (as we'll soon see) how. These distractions will not help you reestablish a new relationship with food, it will only confirm the old relationship (as chances are this is an old habit). You want to be deliberate, not habitual; mindful, not mindless.

4. How? How are you engaging with your food and to the experience of eating? It's not such a silly question. Some people eat to become full or satisfied. But some savor the pleasures of eating, the intermingling of flavors, textures and colors. One may think it's a cultural thing (the French and the Italians in particular are known for the culinary pride), this isn't true. Every culture has important ties to their food. Any American may have the same savory appreciation for a good hamburger that any Frenchman does for a plate of escargot. Food is as central to various Asian cultures as to various Latin

cultures, where the creation of the food is as central to family unity as the eating of the meal itself.

And for a lot of cultures, food is part of the celebration of life.

Is food a celebration, something to be savored in your life, or is it simply a matter of utility?

These two questions address your physical and emotional relationship with your food. Getting in touch with how your food makes you feel can help you tailor your diet to help you optimize your fasts, and thrive in this life.

And whatever you're eating, ask yourself what physiological relationship you have to the food. What reaction does it inspire? A rush of satisfaction and pleasure? Does the food energize, does it leave a bloated or lethargic feeling afterward? What emotional feelings do you have after eating? Satisfaction or guilt? Those are things to keep in mind when understanding and recalibrating your relationship with food.

Mindful Eating Exercises

Here are some exercises to help you recalibrate and reset your relationship with food. These exercises will increase your mindfulness about food and about yourself.

1. The *raisin meditation* is generally done using a raisin, though it can be done with any type of food. You'll soon see why a raisin will work better than, say, a bowl of oatmeal or a plate of spaghetti and meat sauce. This practice seeks to bring complete sensory consciousness of what you're eating. This consciousness extends from the first touch to the aftermath of the last swallow. Though not classically a kind of meditation, it does use the pillars of meditation, which are to focus on one particular thing and blot out thought and feelings about anything else.

This practice is especially potent if you do it while first breaking your fast. Your senses will be at a peak, and you'll be particularly appreciative of what you're focusing on.

First, use your senses to understand the food (here's were a raisin beats spaghetti). Touch the raisin, hold it, pick it up and consider its weight, color, texture. Think about the process it underwent to go from grape to raisin. Think about the crevices in its raisin form, and imagine the smoothness of its grape form. Smell it and consider the smell, it's likely very mild but still familiar, probably from childhood. Note how the smell affects your other senses; does it make you salivate in anticipation? Touch the raisin, consider its density and firmness.

Slowly put the raisin in your mouth. Feel it on your tongue. Test it between your teeth. Bite into it slowly and note the release of flavors, the change in texture. Chew it slowly, concentrate on the rise and fall of the flavor, the deterioration of the grape between your teeth, how little pressure is required.

Swallow with intention and focus, feel the contractions in your throat as the swallowing reflex begins. Follow the raison as it slides down your throat. Feel the rush of chemicals as your body reacts to the new input. It will be subtle, but it will be there. Look for it, note the sensations.

2. When eating, rest your fork between bites. This is a mindfulness exercise which allows you to focus on the food in your mouth instead of the food on your plate. You can focus on the mouthful you're chewing instead of the next one you're about to chew. This encourages the kind of culinary meditation we just looked at, a chance to feel the food in your mouth, note the sensory reactions and the chemical reactions with each bite. Take a moment to note how the flavors are intermingling.

This will also help you to eat slower, which encourages more thorough digestion and continued good health.

This process does make a meal a bit longer in duration, and it may not be practical in social situations. Or it may. If you eat smaller portions (and we all should be) then eating them slower won't leave you lagging behind others with bigger portions and faster eating habits.

You can, however, cultivate generally slower eating habits that force you to pay more attention to your eating patterns.

Best Foods for Breaking a Fast

We've already seen that it's important to eat the right foods, and how to safely break a fast. Now let's look at which healthy foods are best for breaking a fast ... and why. Remember that you're resetting your system, and your new cells will be informed by the newest fuels, or the last things you put into your system. That's why it's important to break your fast with the right foods.

Keep in mind that this is all the more important when breaking long-term fasts. When intermittent fasting, it's less crucial. Though it's still important eat right during intermittent fasting.

Here's a reliable recipe for breaking a fast. Start with a glass of apple cider vinegar and water, and have it before you eat. This stimulates the digestive process. Then have bowl of bone broth, two hard-boiled eggs, iron-rich greens like kale or spinach Try to keep the meal under 500 calories.

But that's a pretty limited choice, and in fact there are a variety of good foods to eat when breaking a fast. I'm not suggesting you feast on a combination of all of them, of course. Use common sense and moderation when breaking your fast.

1. Apple cider vinegar (ACV) is new to the selfcare scene, though it's a remedy which dates back to ancient cultures. ACV's benefits include:

- Levels alkaline PH levels: Though ACV is acidic, it becomes alkaline when consumed
- Kills bad gut bacteria gut: Still, ACV is helpful to good bacteria in the gut
- Stabilizes blood sugar: ACV lowers insulin levels too, and creates a feeling of fullness
- Stimulates digestion
- Improves first-meal digestion

Here's a popular recipe for an ACV drink to enjoy while fasting (not for breaking a fast).

- 10 to 12oz of water
- 2 tablespoons of ACV

- 1/2 teaspoon of Pink Himalayan Salt
- 1/2 teaspoon of cream of tartar
- 2 tablespoons of bottled lime juice or the juice of 1 whole lime
- Stevia to taste

  ACV capsules are also available.

2. Bone broth is popular for its hearty flavor, but that's just the beginning of its benefits, including being:

- Rich in electrolytes (minerals which are dissolved in bodily fluids, creating electrically-charged ions.
- Rich in essential minerals (potassium, magnesium, sodium, and calcium)
- Rich in collagen for healthy bones, nails, and teeth
- Rich in glycine for better sleep, especially during fasting
- Rich in many anti-inflammatory amino acids
- Low in carbohydrates

Bone broth comes as a liquid or powder, both are mixed with a water base.

3. Kale and spinach have come up before, and for good reason. They're rich in essential vitamins and nutrients which are often depleted during fasting, including:

- Vitamin B2, B6
- Vitamin C
- Vitamin A
- Vitamin E
- Vitamin K
- Folate
- Manganese
- Magnesium
- Copper
- Iron
- Potassium
- Calcium

Kale and spinach are good raw, cooked, or whipped in a fruit or veggie smoothie. Either way, the benefits of either one include:

- Helping digestion

- Preventing constipation
- Maintaining blood sugar

4. Eggs are a terrific delivery system for a lot of protein with comparatively little food mass. That protein prevents muscle loss, making it a good way to break a fast. They're also rich in leucine, an amino acid closely related to muscle development. Eggs are also easily digested and rich in protein and can curb the appetite (particularly when hard-boiled).

5. Nuts, chia seeds and others, like flax and helm seeds, pecan and almond. Nuts are popular these days for their potent delivery of essential fats, proteins, nutrients, minerals, and fibers. Chia seeds alone are rich in:

- Phosphorus
- Manganese
- Calcium
- Copper
- Selenium
- Iron

6. Fish and fish broth are great for breaking a fast (the broth especially). But even fish meat will be

a forgiving first meal, and will be a terrific source of unsaturated fat (the healthy kind) with omega 3, vitamin D, and various proteins.

7. Broccoli, cauliflower, and brussels sprouts are cruciferous vegetables, which are rich in nutrients, fiber, and vitamins. Broccoli is the most digestible of these cruciferous vegetables, which are also filled with:

- Vitamin A
- Vitamin C
- Vitamin K
- Vitamin B2
- Vitamin B5
- Vitamin B6
- Vitamin B9
- Iron
- Manganese
- Magnesium

8. Watermelon is rich in fiber, and only a semi-solid food (91% water), both of which make it very easy to digest and which recommend it for breaking a fast.

9. Bananas are filled with healthy carbs (good if you're not doing a keto plan) and are also rich in fiber, potassium, vitamins B6 and C, and can boost blood sugar.

10. Unsweetened Yogurt, Sauerkraut, Kimchi are fermented foods, which are great for good gut bacteria and enzymes lost during a fast. Avoid spicy kimchi recipes.

11. Avocado is the fattiest fruit in the world (the avocado is really just a large berry). It's ideal for breaking a fast because it's low in calories, rich in omega-3 and omega-6 fat, filled with minerals, antioxidants, and vitamins, including:

- Potassium
- Copper
- Folate
- Vitamin B6
- Vitamin K
- Vitamin C
- Vitamin E
- Antothenic acid, which maximizes the use of the others

Note that some people find avocado hard to digest.

Breaking a fast improperly can wreak havoc on the digestive system. When coming off a long-term fast, spend seven days eating these foods before you return to a normal, daily diet. To make that transition easier, eat the ones you enjoy most and can tolerate the easiest. Keep your first post-fast first meal around 500 calories. For the next week, consider your circumstances. If you're more active, consider eggs instead of broth for better muscle growth.

Observing the importance of breaking a fast brings something else to mind, a recurring theme of our practices here, and that's transition. Good change comes gradually, not quickly. If you're fasting long-term or short, if you're exercising or practicing yoga or meditation, for one session or for a whole new lifestyle, transition into and out of these practices slowly. You must precede a fast with a period of light eating (half the duration of the fast) and observe a similar pattern after the fast. Warm up to your exercises and wind down when you're done, same thing with your yoga and meditative practices. And of course, always consult your doctor before engaging in any change in diet or exercise.

And speaking of diet and exercise, this brings us to the elephant in the room, if you'll pardon that turn of phrase. We're talking about fat and cholesterol, the leading reasons for fasting and the maladies fasting seeks to remedy. But any good dietician, yogi, lawyer, football coach, or anyone in a professional capacity will swear by these words: Know your enemy. But is fat really an enemy? Is it the enemy? What about cholesterol? How much do you really know about these things, which course through your body every second of your life? If the answer is not much or not enough, fear not and read on. You're about to know everything you need to move ahead on your journey to physical (and yes, psychological) wellness.

CHAPTER FOUR:
Fats and Cholesterol

Cholesterol

Cholesterol is a waxy substance which collects in the arteries. It is often mistaken for detrimental, but some cholesterol is crucial to good health.

There are two different types of cholesterol; low-density lipoprotein (LDL) and high-density lipoprotein (HDL). LDL is considered the bad cholesterol, HDL is considered the good cholesterol. The reason for this is that HDL carries cholesterol directly to the liver. There is is removed from the bloodstream so it cannot build up in the arteries. LDL delivers cholesterol straight to the arteries. The result may be plaque buildup called atherosclerosis which may cause stroke or heart attack.

Triglycerides are the third major cholesterol component. They are unused calories which the human body stores in the blood as fat. Excessive caloric intake (taking in more calories than you burn) allows triglycerides to collect in the bloodstream, raising the risk of heart attack.

It's important to understand your cholesterol numbers. Over thirty percent of Americans have high LDL (over 100). HDLs, on the other hand, should number no fewer than 40 (for men) or 50 (for women). Healthy triglyceride numbers are 150 or less. Your total cholesterol numbers shouldn't exceed 200.

Fats

Good fats include monounsaturated and polyunsaturated fats. Bad ones include industrial-made trans fats. Saturated fats fall somewhere in the middle. What's the difference? On a chemical level, all fats are structured as a chain of carbon atoms which are bonded to hydrogen atoms. The shape and length of the chain and amount of hydrogen atoms connected are what differentiates one fat molecule from another. Good fats have fewer hydrogen atoms than saturated fats. They're liquid at room temperature, not solid.

So what makes a good fat good and a bad fat bad? Some of the benefits of good, unsaturated fats, acceptable saturated fats, and bad trans fats? Let's take a look at what's good about good fats. The benefits of good (unsaturated) fats include:

- Major source of energy
- Aids vitamin and mineral absorption
- Necessary to building cell membranes
- Essential for muscle movement
- Necessary for blood clotting
- Essential for necessary inflammation

Unsaturated fats

Unsaturated fats are liquid at room temperature. They're beneficial fats which ease inflammation, improve blood cholesterol levels, stabilize the heart rhythms, and which play a number of beneficial roles for the human body. Unsaturated fats are found mostly in plant-based foods like nuts, seeds, and vegetable oils.

There are good fats, which are beneficial to the body, and bad fats, which are detrimental to the body. The two types of "good" unsaturated fats are monounsaturated and Polyunsaturated fats.

The monounsaturated fat came to the fore of dietary studies in the 1960s, revealing how heart rates in the Mediterranean, despite a high-fat diet. This was because the main fat in their diets was olive oil, not saturated animal fat. This is the origin of the Mediterranean diet, which we'll look at in greater detail later in this book.

The Institute of Medicine's recommendations are to use these good fats to replace saturated and trans fats whenever possible. Monounsaturated fats have single carbon-to-carbon double bonds with fewer hydrogen atoms than saturated fat. Foods rich in monounsaturated fats include:

- Nuts (hazelnuts, almonds, and pecans)
- Seeds (sesame and pumpkin seeds)

- Canola oil
- Peanut oil
- Olive oil
- Avocados
- Safflower oil
- Sunflower oil

Polyunsaturated fats are essential fats found in cooking oils. Being essential means they're necessary for normal body function, but they're not made by the body doesn't make them. Polyunsaturated fats are crucial to:

- Build cell membranes
- Covering nerves
- Muscle movement
- Blood clotting
- Necessary internal inflammation

A polyunsaturated fat's carbon chain has two or sometimes more double bonds. Omega-3 fatty acids and omega-6 fatty acids are the two types of polyunsaturated fat. The numbers 3 and 6 refer to the distance between the carbon chain's beginning and the chain's first double bond.

The benefits of omega-3 fatty acids include:

- Possible prevention of stroke and heart disease
- Reduction of blood pressure
- Raising HDL
- Lowering triglycerides
- Control lethal heart rhythms
- Reduction of corticosteroid medications for rheumatoid arthritis
- Reduction of risk of dementia

Omega-6 fatty acids may protect against heart disease and can be found in vegetable oils (safflower, sunflower, soybean, corn, walnut).

Polyunsaturated fats are found in rich supply in:

- Sunflower, soybean, corn, and flaxseed oils
- Flax seeds
- Fish
- Walnut
- Canola oil (for the polyunsaturated fat)

Omega-3 fats are crucial polyunsaturated fats. They have to be introduced into the system, as the human body cannot manufacture or synthesize them. Eating fish two to three times per week is more than sufficient. If you can't stand fish, try these plant-based alternatives: Walnuts, flax seeds, canola and soybean oil. Higher omega-3 levels in the blood are closely associated with a lower risk of death among older adults.

The general population don't get enough unsaturated fats. The recommendation of the American Heart Association is eight to ten percent of a person's daily calories should derive from polyunsaturated fats.

Most people don't eat enough healthful unsaturated fats. The American Heart Association suggests that 8-10 percent of daily calories should come from polyunsaturated fats, and evidence suggests that an increase of up to 15 percent (replacing saturated fat) may lower the risk of heart disease.

Sixty trials conducted by Dutch researchers found that when monounsaturated and polyunsaturated fats replaced carbohydrates, those good fats lowered harmful LDL levels and increased beneficial HDL levels. Another trial proved that swapping carbs for unsaturated (mostly monosaturated) fats lowered blood pressure, improved lipid level, and reduced risk of cardiovascular disease.

Saturated Fats

Saturated refers to the molecular makeup of the fat; the quantity of hydrogen atoms which surround every carbon atom. This chain holds as many as possible, and so it is saturated with hydrogens.

Almost two dozen studies suggest that there is insufficient evidence to prove a connection between saturated fats and heart disease, but there is a connection between polyunsaturated fat and heart disease. Two major studies concluded that replacing saturated fats with polyunsaturated fats such as high-fiber carbs or vegetable oils is the preferred method for reducing heart disease risk, while replacing saturated fat with any highly processed carbohydrate produced the opposite effect.

Plenty of healthy foods (like nuts and chicken) have some saturated fat. But some, less healthy foods (like cheese, beef, and ice cream) have much more saturated fat. It's found principally in animal food products, but some plant-based foods have a lot of saturated fats as well (oils derived from coconut, palm and palm kernel).

While saturated fat is better for you than unsaturated fats, it can still be harmful in excess. Experts suggest less saturated fat should account for no more than ten percent of daily caloric intake. The American Heart Association recommends no more than seven percent.

But replacing saturated fats is one thing, the question is what to replace it with. Refined carbohydrates may lower bad cholesterol (low-density lipoprotein or LDL), but it also lowers good cholesterol (high-density lipoprotein or HDL). It also increases triglycerides, also bad for the heart.

We'll talk more about these things in greater detail shortly.

The biggest sources of saturated fat in the United States diet are:
- Whole- or reduced-fat butter, milk, and dairy desserts
- Pizza and cheese
- Some meats (bacon, sausage, hamburgers, beef)
- Cookies (grain-based sweets)
- Fast-food

Recent studies have disproven the old notions that saturated fat is harmful. Other extensive studies showed no connection between saturated fat intake and either cardiovascular or coronary heart disease. Replacing bad fasts with good can help to prevent the body's resistance to insulin, which is a precursor to diabetes.

Trans Fats

Trans fatty acids (also known as *trans fats*) are created by the process hydrogenation (heating liquid vegetable oils near hydrogen gas). By partially hydrogenating these vegetable oils, the oils become more stable and more likely to resist becoming rancid. The same process may harden the vegetable oil into a solid (shortening and margarine). These partially hydrogenated oils withstand repeated cooling and heating, which makes them perfect for frying.

The trans fat offers no health benefits and there is no recommended safe consumption level. And they're officially banned from use in the United States and other countries. And there is no safe level of consumption.

Trans fats are found in dairy fat and beef fat, but in smaller amounts. They're the worst fat for the blood vessels, heart, and other parts of the body. Other risks of consuming too many trans fats include:

- Elevated bad LDL rates, lowered good HDL rates

- Increased inflammation, implicated in stroke, heart disease, diabetes, various chronic conditions
- Increased insulin resistance

Later in this book, we'll look into exercises and diets, some specific to burning fat. There are yoga practices in this book with the same goal in mind. So let's stay in the laboratory, as it were, before we take all these things out into the field. We've learned a lot, but it's like Albert Einstein said: "The more we learn, the more we realize we do not know." And there's still another big field of study we have to go into. But think of everything you've learned about the different fats and types of cholesterol. Think of the confidence it gives you to prevail over it. Think of how good it feels to use your intellect, the one advantage the human being has over most other animals and even over its own body. The more you learn, the better able you'll be to conquer these once-mystical things. So let's prepare to conquer one of natures great mysteries and one of full-body wellnesses greatest necessities, the keys to the Fountain of Youth.

Hormones.

SECTION 2:
HORMONES AND HORMONAL IMBALANCE

CHAPTER FIVE: Hormones

Hormones are an essential part of the body's chemical system. They travel like messengers through the bloodstream as help organs or tissues function at their best. Where they go and what they do depend on what type of hormones are being generated, and that is decided by the trouble spot in the body. Different hormones provide different functions for different parts of the body.

Several endocrine glands secret these hormones, which are necessary for healthy development, growth, reproduction, and other bodily functions. Here's a handy list and rundown of your top ten essential hormones.

The hormones of thyroid, Triiodothyronine (T3) and Thyroxine (T4), are released by the thyroid gland. These hormones help maintain the body's metabolism, regulate weight, determine energy levels, regulates internal temperature, determined hair and skin health, among others.

Insulin is released by the pancreas, from the abdominal cavity, just behind the stomach. Insulin allows the body to use sugar (or glucose) from carbs for energy to use or store. Insulin helps keep blood sugar levels from getting either too low (hypoglycemia) or too high (hyperglycemia).

Estrogen is a female sexual hormone which is released by the ovaries and is responsible for menstruation, reproduction, and menopause. Too much estrogen is known to increase the risks of uterine and breast cancer, moodiness, depression, and other conditions. Too little estrogen can lead to skin lesions, acne, hair loss, thinning skin, weak fingernails, and other symptoms.

Produced in the ovaries, progesterone is produced in the placenta (when a woman is pregnant) in the ovaries and the adrenal glands. Progesterone regulates and stimulates various female bodily functions, including pregnancy maintenance. Progesterone helps the female body prepare for conception and pregnancy, as well as regulating the monthly menstrual cycle.

Progesterone levels drop when a lack of pregnancy initiates the menstrual cycle. Progesterone plays a big role in human sexual desire.

Prolactin is released by the pituitary gland. It's released after childbirth and it enable a female to lactate and breastfeed. Prolactin levels rise during pregnancy and can boost fertility.

Testosterone is a male sexual hormone. This anabolic (muscle-building) steroid helps build muscle. Testosterone is also key to developing reproductive tissues in the male body, the testes and the prostate. Testosterone also promotes increased muscle mass, bodily hair and other secondary sexual characteristics. Testosterone deficiency may cause frailty and bone loss in men.

Serotonin is a hormone known for rejuvenation, and it's closely associated with memory and learning, sleep and mood regulation, digestion, and muscular development. Serotonin deficiency is associated with migraines, depression, insomnia, weight gain, carbohydrate craving. Too much serotonin may cause agitation, sedation, and confusion.

The adrenal gland produces Cortisol, the hormone which maintains overall good health and energy. Cortisol controls psychological and physical stress. In times of stress, cortisol increases blood pressure, heart rate, and respiration. But consistently high cortisol levels may cause high blood pressure, ulcer, anxiety, high cholesterol levels. Cortisol deficiency is known to cause alcoholism, chronic fatigue syndrome, and other conditions.

The adrenal gland secretes adrenaline, known as an emergency hormone. Adrenaline is released to counter stress. It dilates blood vessels to the brain and heart.

Somatotropin is also called the growth hormone. Somatotropin is a protein hormone which has 190 amino acids that are synthesized by celled known as *somatotrophs*. Somatotropin stimulates growth, cell regeneration and reproduction, and boosts metabolism.

Here's a supplementary list of other hormones and what they do for your body.

Adrenocorticotropic hormone (ACTH) stimulates cortisol production.

Aldosterone is central to sound cardiovascular health, and it may be a cause of endocrine hypertension.

Angiotensin is a common name for four hormones and play an important role in blood pressure regulation. Learn how this hormone affects many aspects of your health and how to keep it in balance.

Angiotensin is actually the common name for four different hormones. It plays a crucial role in regulating blood pressure.

Anti-Müllerian Hormone (AMH) aids in fertility and reproductive health in human females.

Calcitonin, among the body's most critical hormones, controls potassium and calcium levels.

Cholecystokinin is a hormone best known for helping to improve digestion.

Dehydroepiandrosterone (DHEA) is a precursor hormone with little biological efficacy until converted into other hormones and used for human reproduction.

Dihydrotestosterone stimulates development of various male physical characteristics. Dihydrotestosterone levels are contingent on testosterone levels.

Erythropoietin is a hormone which supports red blood cell production.

The strongest of the three estrogens, Estradiol is important to the female reproductive system. It's the most common type of estrogen for women who are of childbearing age.

Estriol, by comparison, is a minor estrogen hormone which promotes uterus growth. Estriol prepares a human female for giving birth.

Estrone is the third type of estrogen and it's the only estrogen made by the body makes after menstrual periods stop (menopause).

The hormone gastrin governs gastric acid release. Gastrin breaks proteins.

Ghrelin is a digestive hormone which controls appetite.

The pancreas produces the peptide hormone glucagon in order to regulate glucose in the bloodstream.

That's not to be confused with the glucagon-like peptide 1 (GLP-1). This hormone, produced in the small intestine, prevents glucagon production, resulting in lower blood sugar levels. GLP-1 also stimulates insulin production.

Gonadotrophin-releasing hormone (GnRH) secretes reproductive hormones including follicle-stimulating hormone (FSH) and luteinizing hormone (LH).

The human chorionic gonadotropin (HcG) hormone is crucial to the early stages of pregnancy.

Made in the hypothalamus, the hormone kisspeptin initiates the release of other hormones.

Leptin helps control weight and appetite.

Luteinizing hormone (LH) controls female and male reproductive systems.

Melanocyte-stimulating hormone (MSH) protects skin from ultraviolet rays, promotes pigmentation development, and controls appetite.

Melatonin regulates the wake and sleep cycle and has become popular as a sleep aid.

The hormone and neurotransmitter norepinephrine breaks down fat, increases heart rate and blood pressure, and more.

Oxytocin is vital for labor and childbirth, breastfeeding, social behaviors, and bonding.

The parathyroid hormone affects calcium levels in the intestines, kidney, and naturally in the bones.

Peptide YY is produced to signal that you're full and have eaten enough. It's produced in the small intestine.

Prostaglandins aid in healing tissue damage or fighting infection.

Relaxin is produced in the female body when she prepares to deliver a newborn.

Somatostatin (SST), a growth hormone, inhibits the secretion of various other hormones.

Thyroxine aids heart and muscle functioning, digestion, bone maintenance, and brain development, and bone maintenance.

Vitamin D is a hormone which promotes bone growth and calcium absorption and bone growth.

Well, now you've met the rogue's gallery of hormones. Some are lusty rascals, some are young pup eager to grow. They're not easy to control, but you cannot (and probably wouldn't want to) live without them. But knowing, in this case, is only half the battle. Like a crowd of ill-tempered children, they have to be nurtured and looked after. They can quickly become imbalanced, and that can wreak absolute havoc. There are ways they can do this, and ways to regain control and re-achieve a lost balance. It's not that hard, but it takes mindfulness and deliberate action, as you'll see.

CHAPTER SIX:
Hormonal Imbalance

This is where hormones go from the being the body's best friends to its worst enemies. Hormonal imbalance can change the whole chemical balance of the body and instigate all manner of dangerous conditions. But how do you know if you have a hormonal imbalance? And if you do, how do you know how to correct it?

Why, you read on, of course.

Signs or Symptoms of a Hormonal Imbalance

We've already seen how hormones play a crucial part in the overall health of the human body. But there's a variety of hormones which perform a variety of functions, as we've already seen. So naturally there are a variety of symptoms and signs of hormonal imbalance.

Some of the most common hormonal imbalances which affect both women and men may cause any of these symptoms or signs:

- Fatty hump on the back between the shoulder blades
- weight gain
- sudden, unexplained weight loss
- muscle weakness
- fatigue
- stiffness, swelling, or pain in the joint
- muscle aches, tenderness, and stiffness
- sweating
- increased or decreased heart rate
- greater sensitivity to heat or cold
- frequent urination
- constipation or more frequent bowel movements
- increased hunger
- increased thirst
- depression
- decreased sex drive
- blurred vision

- nervousness, irritability, or anxiety
- Thinning or brittle hair
- Infertility
- Sleeplessness
- Stress
- Dry skin
- Puffy or rounded face
- purple or pink stretch marks

Signs or Symptoms in Females

Reproductive-age females often endure polycystic ovary syndrome (PCOS), a common hormonal imbalance. The normal female hormonal cycle also changes naturally according to these states of life:
- puberty
- pregnancy
- breastfeeding
- menopause

Symptoms of hormonal imbalance which are specific to females include:

- heavy or irregular periods (including stopped or missed or frequent periods)
- hirsutism (excessive hair on the chin, face, chest, or other parts of the body)
- acne on the chest, upper back, or face, chest, or upper back
- skin tags
- hair loss
- skin darkening (along neck creases, under the breasts, in the groin)
- vaginal atrophy
- vaginal dryness
- night sweats
- pain during sex
- headaches
- Menstruation won't begin
- Breast tissue won't develop
- Growth rate remains static

Symptoms and Signs in Males

Hormonal imbalance can be just as complicated and varied for men as for women.

Insufficient testosterone and other imbalances can have a variety of symptoms and signs, including:
- Breast tenderness
- Gynecomastia (development of breast tissue)
- Erectile dysfunction (ED)
- Loss of muscle mass
- decrease in bodily and facial hair growth
- Loss of bone mass (osteoporosis)
- Hot flashes
- difficulty concentrating

Boys with hormonal imbalance may experience:
- High-pitched voice
- Lack of muscle mass development
- Sparse bodily hair growth
- Impaired testicular or penile growth
- Excessive growth of legs and arms, relative to the torso
- Gynecomastia

Causes of Hormonal Imbalance

With the wide variety of hormones and functions, their causes are also widely varied, including:
- Prescription medications
- Hormone therapy
- Cancer treatments (like chemotherapy)
- Benign or cancerous tumors
- Eating disorders
- Pituitary tumors
- Stress
- Trauma or injury

The following conditions may originate with hormonal imbalances and may lead to other imbalances.
- Diabetes insipidus
- Diabetes (type 1 and type 2)
- Hyperthyroidism (overactive thyroid)
- Hypothyroidism (an underactive thyroid)
- hyperthyroidism, or an overactive thyroid
- hyperfunctioning thyroid nodules

- Hypogonadism
- Thyroiditis
- Congenital adrenal hyperplasia (causing low levels of aldosterone and cortisol)
- Cushing syndrome (or high levels of cortisol)
- Addison's disease

Causes Which are Unique to Women

A lot of causes of female hormonal imbalance relate to the reproductive hormones, and the common causes are:
- Premature menopause (primary ovarian insufficiency)
- Menopause
- Pregnancy
- PCOS
- Breastfeeding
- Birth control pills

Tests for Hormonal Imbalance

Because the variety of hormonal functions is so wide, there's no single test for hormonal imbalance. But a trip to your physician is a good place to start. Be prepared with a list of symptoms and a timeline and any external factors like stress, medications, or supplements you may be taking. Be prepared to answer the following questions:

- How often do symptoms occur?
- How do you relieve symptoms?
- Have you gained or lost weight recently?
- Is there more stress in your life?
- Are you trying to get pregnant?
- Was your last period regular and on time?
- Do you have ED?
- Do you experience vaginal pain or dryness during sex?

Expect a blood test to check thyroid health and levels of testosterone, cortisol, and/or estrogen.

A pelvic exam and pap smear may be recommended for female patients to check for unusual cysts, tumors, or lumps. For men, the scrotum may be observed for abnormalities or lumps.

An ultrasound test uses sonic waves to retrieve images of ovaries, the uterus, testicles, pituitary gland, or thyroid. uses sound waves to look inside your body.

You may also try a variety of at-home testing kids, available for a wide spectrum of conditions. These tests use blood or saliva to measure key thyroid hormones, sex hormones like testosterone and progesterone, and cortisol.

Some of these tests require the user to send a sample away in the mail. Results are often returned between five and ten days. Most, but not all, of these tests are FDA-approved.

Treatments for Hormonal Imbalance

As you might have guessed, treatments for hormonal imbalance are as varied as the causes of those imbalances. Here are few common treatment options!

Estrogen therapy is popular for hot flashes and other symptoms of menopause. This treatment employs small supplemental doses of estrogen. This kind of hormone replacement therapy (HRT) should be discussed with a medical professional.

Vaginal estrogen may be applied as a cream, administered in a tablet or in an insertable ring in the case of pain or dryness during sex. This local treatment sidesteps the risks of systemic estrogen, which travels through the bloodstream to its target organ.

Hormonal birth control works by helping to regulate the menstrual cycle. Types of hormonal birth control include:
- Birth control patch
- Birth control shot
- Birth control pill
- Intrauterine device (IUD)
- Vaginal ring

It may also help improve acne and reduce extra hair on the face and body.

Anti-androgen medications are often effective. Androgens, male sex hormones, are present in women as well as men. Women with high levels of androgens may prefer medication to block the androgens' effects, which may include:

- Facial hair growth
- Hair loss
- Acne

Testosterone theory introduces supplements to reduce symptoms of low testosterone in males. This type of therapy, available in a patch, a gel, or by injection, is popular in cases of delayed puberty.

Thyroid hormone therapy introduces supplements of a synthetic thyroid hormone called levothyroxine (comprised of Unithroid, Synthroid, and Levoxyl) may achieve hormonal balance.

Metformin is a medication for type 2 diabetes which has been helpful for some women presenting symptoms of PCOS. The FDA-unapproved treatment may encourage ovulation and lower androgen levels.

Addyi (flibanserin) and Vyleesi (bremelanotide) are the only FDA-approved medications for low sexual desire in women who are premenopausal. Vyleesi is a self-administered injectable. Addyi comes in a pill form.

Those drugs are associated with side effects like blood pressure changes and severe nausea. in blood pressure.

Vaniqa (eflornithine) is a cream prescribed for excessive female facial hair. It slows new growth but does not remove existing hair.

Natural Supplements and Remedies

There are no natural supplements proven to treat menopause or the hormonal imbalance that goes along with it. But there are supplements for the various symptoms. Melatonin may help with sleep, Coenzyme Q-10 (CoQ-10) and glutathione are excellent cellular supplements. Resveratrol and the previously mentioned curcumin are powerful anti-inflammatories.

A lot of supplements have plant-based hormones which chemically resemble a human body's hormones. Whether these are more effective than direct hormone replacement theory isn't well-known.

Yoga and meditation are two ways a lot of people approach their hormonal imbalances, and we'll take a closer look at them a little later in this book.

Lifestyle Changes for Hormone Management

Other holistic, non-pharmaceutical approaches to hormonal imbalances include changes in lifestyle:

Lose weight. Sources report that a ten-percent reduction in total body weight may help make menstrual periods more regular and it may also increase the chances of getting pregnant. In men, weight loss can improve proper erectile function.

Eat well. A balanced diet is important to overall good health.

Decrease vaginal discomfort by using moisturizers and lubes which are free of glycerin, parabens, and/or petroleum.

Avoid hot flashes by identifying common triggers, such as spicy foods, warm temperatures, or hot beverages.

Remove unwanted or excess body or facial hair. Laser hair removal, electrolysis, or hair removal creams are popular.

Other Hormonal Imbalances

Acne is associated with hormonal imbalance as well, which creates excessive oil production.

Hormonal imbalance and weight gain are closely associated, as hormones play such an integral role in metabolism. Cushing syndrome and other hormone disorders often cause weight gain and even obesity thanks to the elevated levels of cortisol in the blood. Increased appetite and fat storage are the natura results of high cortisol levels. Severe hypothyroidism may likewise lead to weight gain.

Diet and exercise remain the best way to deal with weight, but intermittent fasting is a powerful tool as well, as we've seen.

So there are ways to control and rebalance certain hormones. Exercises and yoga practices we'll look at do the same, and we'll go through them in considerable detail. For now, let's take a closer look at hormones, because they have a strong grounding in heredity. Hormones are not strictly a matter of age, diet, or environment. They're as much about the past, even the distant past, as they are about the present or the future. And if you're going to truly be in the optimal control of your hormones, it's important to know when and if you can't control them at all; and if you can, how.

CHAPTER SEVEN:
Hormones and Heredity

The word *hormone* derives from the Ancient Greek word for *impetus*. And that only makes sense, as hormones are the driving force of growth and chemical behavior, mood changing, mating, eating, drinking, fleeing and fighting.

And while there are numerous connections between hormonal imbalance and lifestyle influences, including medicinal and dietary. We've looked at some ways to treat these imbalances, many behavioral and chemical. But it's not all about lifestyle or intake. There are strong connections to heredity, and this must be considered when dealing with hormonal imbalances and how to deal with them.

Let's look at this fairly complex medical web of nature and nurture in a fairly straightforward way. Genes code for hormones and hormone receptors as well as hormone precursors. Genes also contain the necessary codes for hormonal synthesis, bodily transport and, finally, elimination. Science has already identified a lot of these specific genes as they relate to hormonal signaling.

The CRH gene, for example, codes for the corticotrophin-releasing hormone, in this case in the service of cortisol release in response to stress.

For depression and cognitive ability, genetic differences play a big part. We're not sure precisely how, other than allowing for intergenerational temperamental tendencies. Likewise, we know hormones operate on a genetic basis, but we can't say exactly how we can manipulate those genes to prevent the concurrent hormonal imbalances.

Is there a connection between hormone-related genes and related behaviors? Recent studies on alcohol use indicate that a specific gene, Srd5a1, contributes to the synthesis of a neuroactive steroid. Other papers used family designed in examining links between genetic (though latent) risks for psychopathology and hormonal processes. For example, biological mothers reporting substance abuse were linked with their children's cortisol levels early in the day. Another published paper investigated the connection between genetic risk for substance abuse in adolescence and certain genetic influences on healthy pubertal development.

And it's not just a one-way street. Genes do code for hormones, and hormones, in return, regulate genes. Steroid hormones (estradiol, cortisol, testosterone, and progesterone) ahdere to intracellular receptors which regulate the gene's expression.

It leads one to ask whether hormonal changes (such as in puberty or menopause) can suppress or activate genetic influences on a behavioral phenotype. The second question is whether changes in gene expression is involved with that influence. Which is in charge, genetics or behavior?

In short, hormones and genetics simply interact around these forces, each playing their part as required. It's more of an interplay than a cause/effect relationship.

Genetic Syndromes / Endocrine Diseases

Genetic syndromes are not necessarily connected to hormonal disorders. They are medical conditions which are caused by genetically inherited gene mutations. They are passed down from generation to generation. It's very rare that these are related to endocrine organs, occurring only once for every half-million to million cases.

For example, the majority of parathyroid and thyroid diseases have no genetic component. Patients are asked, but report no family history of the diseases.

On the other hand, roughly 33% of diagnosed pheochromocytoma (tumor of the adrenal medulla) cases are currently believed to be genetic and inherited. The most commonly associated genetic conditions include:

- Multiple endocrine neoplasia (MEN) type 2
- von Hippel-Lindau syndrome
- Neurofibromatosis type 1
- Familial paraganglioma syndrome

Multiple Endocrine Neoplasia (MEN) Syndromes

Multiple Endocrine Neoplasia (MEN) syndromes are inherited. A mutated gene creates malignant and benign neuroendocrine tumors. Since it is the endocrine glands which can overproduce hormones and present as symptoms. Early diagnosis and quick treatment always recommended to treat MEN syndromes.

To better understand these syndromes, let's take a closer look at the variants: MEN-I, MEN-IIA, MEN-IIB, familial medullary thyroid cancer (itself a variant of MEN-IIA) and MEN-IV.

MEN-I: In multiple endocrine neoplasia (MEN) I, one or more glands develop adenoma (tumor) or excess normal tissue (hyperplasia). MEN-I generally strikes the pancreas, the parathyroid, and the pituitary, glands. It sometimes strikes the thyroid and adrenal glands. These endocrine glands produce and secrete hormones into the lymph or blood systems.

Symptoms of this syndrome include:
- Peptic ulcer disease
- Symptoms of high serum calcium or kidney stones
- Symptoms of pituitary difficulties, including headaches
- Low blood sugar
- Hypoglycemia
- Hypercalcemia (pituitary dysfunction)
- Abdominal pain
- Aching, burning, hunger discomfort in the lower chest or upper abdomen which is relieved by milk, food, or antacids.
- Black stools
- Vomiting and nausea
- Feeling bloated after meals
- Headache
- Weakness
- Anxiety
- Lack of coordination
- Vision problems
- Confusion or mental changes

- Coma from untreated hypoglycemia
- Muscle pain
- Loss of appetite
- Sensitivity to cold
- Fatigue
- Low blood pressure
- Unintentional weight loss
- Loss of pubic and bodily hair
- Infertility, cessation of menses, failure to lactate in women
- Loss of facial or body hair, decreased sexual interest in men

Treatment depends upon which glands are affected. Surgical removal of the gland is often the favored treatment. A bromocriptine may be recommended in the case of a pituitary adenoma. Hormone replacement therapy is often recommended after a gland has been removed.

As to a prognosis, every case has to be taken on its own. Parathyroid and pituitary tumors are often benign, though malignancies do occur. It's easier to treat the symptoms, such as those of peptic ulcer, hypercalcemia, hypoglycemia, and pituitary dysfunction.

MEN-II: Multiple endocrine neoplasia II (MEN II) presents as a thyroid cancer type and is accompanied by a recurring cancer striking the adrenal glands.

MEN-II is caused by a mutation in the gene RET. It presents as multiple tumors which do not necessarily appear at the same time. It affects women and men equally and may strike at any age. There are actually two variants of MEN-II, designated A and B. MEN-IIA may cause hyperparathyroidism, medullary thyroid cancer, and pheochromocytoma. MEN-IIB is more closely associated with neuromas (bumps on the tongue and lips), but also causes medullary thyroid cancer and pheochromocytoma.

Common symptoms of MEN-II include:
- Heart palpitations
- Severe headache
- Rapid heart rate
- Chest pain
- Sweating

- Abdominal pain
- Irritability
- Nervousness
- Weight loss
- Cough
- Cough with blood
- Diarrhea
- Back pain
- Fatigue
- Increased thirst
- Increased urinary output
- Nausea
- Loss of appetite
- Depression
- Muscular weakness
- Personality changes

Treatments for sufferers of MEN-II include surgery, needed to remove the pheochromocytoma and the medullary carcinoma of the thyroid. Treating medullary carcinoma must include the removal of the thyroid gland and (surrounding) lymph nodes.

After surgery, hormone replacement therapy is often suggested.

As this is also an inherited disease, family members should be screened for the related RET mutation.

The prognosis, once again, must be mixed. Pheochromocytoma is often benign. The accompanying medullary carcinoma of the thyroid, however, and which characterizes this condition, is a very aggressive malignant cancer. Early diagnosis and successful surgery often leads to cure.

MEN-IV: Multiple endocrine neoplasia type 4 (MEN4) is a very rare form of the syndrome, characterized by anterior pituitary and parathyroid tumors. MEN-IV may be associated with renal, adrenal, and reproductive organ tumors.

Succinate Dehydrogenase (SDH) syndromes: The SDH is a gene which helps to suppress tumor growth. A mutation in this gene means a greater likelihood of pheochromocytomas and paragangliomas (a tumor which forms near nerves and blood vessels outside the adrenal glands).

Tumors may cause anxiety, stress, and a fight-or-flight response.

Von Hippel-Lindau syndrome is caused by a mutated VHL gene which prevents tumor growth. Roughly 10-34% of VHL syndrome patients may develop paragangliomas or pheochromocytomas, but they may also develop hemoangioblastomas (benign tumors in the linings of certain blood vessels), retinal angiomas (benign lesions with visual and systemic implications), neuroendocrine tumors of the pancreas and renal cell cancers.

Neurofibromatosis type I is resultant of a mutated NF1 gene, which inhibits tumor growth. Patients may develop numerous benign tumors of the skin and nerves and abnormal patches of skin pigmentation. Cognitive abnormalities are common among sufferers, who are at risk for soft tissue sarcomas and other certain cancers. Over five percent of NF-1 sufferers also develop paragangliomas and pheochromocytomas.

And that brings us to the end of our studious investigation of the biology, chemistry, historical, and even psychological aspects of optimal autophagy and total wellness. Armed with this information, you're now ready to play a more physical role and put your new knowledge into effect. You've got the data, now it's time to use it.

So prepare yourself for the next stage in your journey to total wellness. It's already been a challenge, introducing words and concepts which were no doubt intimidating. You have reread passages or chapters, or you may reread them in the future. Good, that's how this book is meant to be used. What lay ahead are also things which are meant to be revisited; exercises, yoga practices, meditations, and of course diets and detoxing.

The first step is detoxing, cleaning out the system before and as you rebuild a healthier one by the process of autophagy.

SECTION 3: DETOXING

CHAPTER EIGHT: Cleanses and Other Detox Programs

The most popular (not-fasting) way to detox is a cleanse, and there are a variety of ways to do that. But before we get into cleanses a bit more deeply, let's take a quick look at some of the more drastic alternatives.

Flushing

Flushing has become a popular way of cleansing the system. But instead of doing so gradually, by means of a fast or even a cleanse, some choose to flush their bodies out. This has benefits and drawbacks and a variety of in-home and clinical applications.

Enemas are a common, inexpensive, and do-it-yourself, at-home way to cleanse your bowel and gut. Kits can be bought at virtually any pharmacy or drug store or even major grocery store.

There are a variety of different enema approaches. The main difference comes down to the solution which is used in the process. The solution will depend on the particular malady which creates the need for the enema in the first place. These may include:

- Water (general blockage)
- Saltwater (constipation)
- Coffee (use only mold-free and organic beans)
- Garlic (parasites and candida)
- Chamomile (cleansing and healing)
- Apple cider vinegar (healing)
- Probiotics (inflammation of the gut)
- Lemon juice (pH balance)
- Mineral oil (constipation)
- Soap (constipation)

Caveats of Enemas

At-home enemas do have some benefits; affordability, convenience, privacy. But there are possible drawbacks.

Coffee and lemon juice are highly acidic. They can damage intestinal lining. Tools which aren't sufficiently cleaned may cause bowel infections. Enemas eliminate good bacteria along with the bad, which leads to further digestive disruptions. Using too much solution can cause stretching and tearing of the bowel. Nausea and vomiting are common during or after a cleanse. Overuse of enemas may weaken the bowel muscles and disrupt natural bowel movements, creating a dependence.

The Coffee Enema

As long as we're going deep into this subject (don't judge me), let's take a look at one of the most popular at-home enemas, the coffee enema.

Drinking coffee remains a controversial practice. While done in various corners of the world, the benefits and drawbacks remain in question. It almost seems to go in and out of style depending on the most recent studies. Because it's so popular and widely consumed, it gets studied a lot. Over the years, coffee has been blamed for liver damage and praised for it benefits to the liver. It's been chastised as a drug and lauded as a alternative beverage to a number of other, more addictive substances like alcohol. It's known to be a powerful antioxidant.

And injecting a coffee solution into your colon has been called a great way to cleanse the lower intestines. Coffee enemas sound like some new(ish) fad, but they've been in use since the turn of the Twentieth century. At the time they were useful to speed healing after surgeries and to combat accidental poisoning. By the 1950s, coffee enemas became standard practice in cancer treatments. Only now are they returning to popularity for a variety of ailments which do not respond properly to prescription medications or traditional treatments.

Coffee's properties as an antioxidant makes it a good choice for a cleanse, as do other beneficial compounds such as palmitate, cafestol theobromine, kahweol, theophylline, and of course caffeine. They're also known to have positive effects on internal inflammation, often a digestive problem requiring an enema.

Coffee enemas have been shown to have these benefits:
- Flushing out heavy metals, bacteria, yeast, fungus from the digestive system
- Cleansing the colon and the liver
- Lowering inflammation
- Restore bowel function
- Relax bowel muscles
- Opens blood vessels
- Opens bile ducts
- Increase bile production
- Increase energy levels of bowel function
- Healing bowel disorders
- Stimulates glutathione S-transferase in the liver
- Repair digestive tissue
- Cleanse the liver
- Improving blood circulation
- Increasing immunity

- Clean out diverticulitis
- Help cellular regeneration
- Relieve digestive issues (bloating, constipation, nausea, and cramping)
- Improve gut health
- Improve moods and energy levels and moods

And so, they're often used to help manage such conditions as:

- Parasites
- Cancer
- Overdoses
- Liver dysfunction
- Candida virus
- Constipation
- IBS (irritable bowel syndrome)
- Various digestive disorders

As with any enema, it's recommended to perform it immediately after a bowel movement. Some recommend an activated carbon charcoal binder both before and after the enema to bind the toxins before release for more efficient elimination.

Enemas are recommended once weekly. Patients healing from digestive disorders may do one per day. Very ill patients, such as those recovering from cancer, may have several per day.

Coffee Enema Dangers and Side Effects

Studies haven't shown too many verified ill-effects of coffee enemas. But their effectiveness will vary from person to person and from case to case. All enemas do carry some risk, as we've discussed: colon tearing, dehydration, electrolyte imbalance, dizziness, and weakness. They're not recommended for children or pregnant women nor for anybody who is allergic to coffee or caffeine.

Clinical Colon Therapy

Besides at-home enemas, there are clinical approaches, including a variety of colon therapy clinics. Some are smaller, meant for quick visits. Others have more of a spa atmosphere, and include baths, massages, and appropriate nourishment. More elaborate overnight colon spas are around too, which provide a two-day cleanse with a (sometimes) private room overnight. My brother used to go to such a place quite often; I used to call it *Flushing Meadows*.

Cleanses

Cleanses are just about the most popular method of detoxing at home. And once detoxes became so widespread, they also became varied, with different new trends and discoveries creating new cleansing recipes and techniques. Some make wild claims, some can actually make good on those promises. So let's take a look at the spectrum of detox regiments, including diets, drinks, and powders … oh my!

It's important to note that these cleanses are so new and inventive, many have not been clinically tested. There may be anecdotal evidence (informally reported), but there is little in the way of clinical trials. And these are regiments, not copyrighted formulas, so they don't get or seek FDA (Food & Drug Administration) approval. So take these regiments with a grain of salt.

The reputed benefits of detoxification include weight loss, improved energy, relief from headaches and muscle aches, fatigue and constipation.

On the other hand, the human body has ways of detoxifying itself, including urinating, defecating, sweating. The digestive tract, liver and kidneys, all break down toxins and prepare them to be eliminated.

But proponents of these cleanses will tell you that the body's natural processes are no longer sufficient to keep up with our modern world and the considerable uptick in toxins we now have to endure. Our bodies haven't changed much since the paleolithic era. But in the last century or so, the industrial age brought pollution like the world as we knew it had never seen. The atomic and nuclear ages brought even more toxicity to our oceans, our rainwater, our soil. Practices like natural gas mining (also known as *fracking*) and disasters like the British Petroleum oil spill in the Gulf of Mexico have made our environment radically toxic. Add to that the shift in our dietary habits over that same century. This century saw the rise of processed foods, sugar substitutes, genetically modified foods. Steroids artificially fattened animals for maximum profitability. Insecticides became a staple of industrial farming, which also robbed the soil of the nutrients which vegetables and fruits require. Tobacco was modified with chemicals for a variety of diabolical reasons.

Our paleolithic systems were never designed to process such an array of toxins, so the liver and kidneys can't be relied upon to do the job. Hence, the need to cleanse. And not only should a cleanse eliminate collected toxins, it would therefore make way for the body to intake new nutrients in their place.

The basic way a detox works is to eliminate specific foods and food groups. This allows the system to stop processing those toxins and heal from the corrosive effects of toxins on the body. The solid foods are replaced, usually with drinks comprised of various natural ingredients, each recipe designed with a certain approach to the body. Some of these ingredients include lemon, cayenne pepper, maple syrup, green tea, or fresh vegetable and fruit juices. Cleanses may last from a single day to an entire month.

Caveats of Cleansing

As we've pointed out, there is little in the way of clinical trails tracing the effectiveness of cleansing. Unless you're suffering from gastroparesis or Crohn's disease, skipping foods in unlikely to generate any healing, according to doctors. The fiber in vegetables and fruits slows digestion and helps the body absorb nutrients and remove toxins through the stool. The digestive tract utilizes fiber's probiotics to nourish the intestines with bacteria, needed for a strong immune system.

And, as we've noted, weight loss from cleanses (as from long-term fasting) is usually temporary. It's mostly water weight and stored stool, which is naturally replaced. The rest of that weight is basically stored carbohydrates, and a dietary change would be needed to prevent that from recurring. Most dietary regiments include some carbohydrates, and exercise is necessary to prevent carb storage.

Athletes should avoid cleansing, as they actually use the stored carbohydrates their bodies carry. Athletic bodies don't use the keto dietary method of using fat as fuel, as their bodies often don't have that much stored fat.

In fact, experts recommend that nobody who is fasting should exercise at the same time. Nor should athletes cleanse while recovering from sports injuries, for the same reason. The body needs those nutrients.

Pros and Cons of Detoxing

Cleansing requires some commitment; of time, of money, of your personal health. You're well-advised to know the pros and cons of your new exploit. Just to remind you; consult with your doctor before changing your diet or exercise protocol.

The pros of cleansing include an increase of minerals and vitamins from fresh juice supplements, and new insight into food sensitivities by process of elimination and reintroduction

The cons of cleansing include lack of energy and disruption of blood glucose levels and disruption of the metabolic rate. Frequent bowel movements and gastrointestinal distress are also common. These diets are also protein deficient. And, as we've discussed, cleansing makes exercise unwise, and this can cause atrophy, sloth, ultimate weight gain, and other related conditions.

Tips for Detoxing

No matter which type of cleanse or detox you prefer, these tips will maximize the efficiency of your campaign and ensure a healthier transition to a healthier lifestyle.

1. Limit your alcoholic intake. The liver processes about ninety percent of alcohol, and when the liver enzymes do metabolize alcohol it becomes acetaldehyde, which is a chemical known to cause cancer. The liver then coverts that toxin to the harmless acetate, later eliminated from the body. Excessive alcoholic intake damages the liver, making it unable to process acetaldehyde to acetate, leading to various cancers (including liver cancer). Fatty buildup, scarring, and inflammation are other was alcohol can damage the liver.

Health authorities recommend no more than two drinks a day (for men) and one drink a day (for women) and two for men. This isn't a recommendation to start drinking if you don't drink now, however.

2. Get more sleep. The body gets a lot done when it is at rest, including various detoxification processes. It's good for the brain and for the psyche as well. During a fast, getting adequate sleep is especially important.

The brain reorganizes and recharges during sleep, but it also removes toxic byproducts. One of these is the protein beta-amyloid, a major factor Alzheimer's disease development.

Lack of sleep may also contribute to:

- Anxiety
- Stress
- Heart disease
- High blood pressure
- Obesity
- Type 2 diabetes

Experts recommend seven to nine hours of sleep per night.

A number of things may interrupt or prevent sleep, including erratic scheduling, light from electronic devices, caffeine, stress, and anxiety.

3. Drink more water. Water has several health benefits which are especially crucial during a cleanse. The benefits of drinking more water include:

- Thirst quenching
- Body temperature regulation
- Joint lubrication
- Digestive aid
- Nutrient absorption
- Natural detoxification
- Waste product removal

Experts recommend and 91 oz (2.7 liters) for women and 125 oz (3.7 liters) for men, though this may vary depending on activity level, diet, and environment.

4. Limit sugar intake. Excessive sugar intake is closely linked to obesity, cancer, heart disease, and diabetes. These are the diseases often preventing the body's ability to detoxify by damaging the organs responsible for detoxification, like the kidneys and liver.

5. Increase antioxidant intake. Oxidation is the breakdown of matter by loss of molecular electrons. If you've ever seen metal rusting, you've witnessed the oxidation process. And this happens inside the human body as well. Molecules lose electrons and become free radicals. While some free radicals are beneficial, as in the digestive process, an excess of free radicals can do damage the body in various ways, including tearing at the inner walls of veins and arteries. Pollutants, alcohol, the chemicals found in tobacco smoke, and poor diet can create excessive free radicals. Free radicals are associated with deadly diseases and conditions including heart disease, dementia, asthma, liver disease, and various cancers.

6. Antioxidants introduce new electrons to correct the free radicals and make them fully functioning molecules again.

Popular antioxidants include:

- Vitamins A, C, E
- Selenium
- Lycopene

- Lutein
- Zeaxanthin

These are commonly found in:

- Fruits
- Berries
- Vegetables
- Cocoa
- Spices
- Nuts
- Coffee
- Green tea

7. Listen to Your Gut. No, we don't mean your gut instinct, but your actual gut. This part of your body is crucial to your overall health, as it is central to digestion and vital to detoxification.

And central to good gut health are good bacteria called prebiotics. These produce short-chain fatty acids, nutrients which are very beneficial to overall health.

But antibiotics, poor dental hygiene, and quality of diet can create an imbalance between good and bad bacteria. This may weaken the detoxification and immune systems and may increase the risk of inflammation and disease.

Foods that are rich in prebiotics include:

- Artichokes
- Tomatoes
- Bananas
- Onions
- Asparagus
- Garlic
- Oats

8. Limit salt intake: Too much salt causes the body to retain fluids. This can be complicated by conditions of the liver or kidneys, or in the case of insufficient water consumption. Given insufficient water and too much salt, the body creates and secretes an antidiuretic hormone which prevents urination. This can cause bloating and general discomfort. Increased water intake actually helps flush out water weight caused by too much salt by instigating urination, washing out the salt as well.

The effects of too much sodium can be counterbalanced by eating potassium-rich foods such as:

- Bananas
- Spinach
- Kidney beans
- Squash
- Potatoes

9. Reduce inflammation. Inflammation does have its proper place, such as wound recovery. But excessive inflammation of internal tissues can contribute to a number of life-threatening conditions, including cancers, high blood pressure, heart disease, stroke, and type 2 diabetes.

Exercise can be tricky during a cleanse (and is to be avoided during a fast) but it can help control inflammation. Experts suggest between 150–300 minutes (per regular dietary week) of moderate exercise (like brisk walking) or 75–150 minutes (per regular dietary week) of vigorous physical activity (like running).

10. Use more spices: Consider eating and cooking with sulfur-rich foods like broccoli, eggs, onions and garlic. These promote glutathione production in the body and help the body excrete heavy metals such as cadmium. Glutathione is a master antioxidant. Chlorella is an algae which helps eliminate toxins such as heavy metals. Cilantro also enhances toxic excretion, particular heavy metals, insecticides, and phthalates.

11. Use natural cleansers: Baking soda and vinegar are just as effective as commercial cleansers and lack a lot of the harmful chemicals.

Let's take a closer look at these chemicals and the risks they pose.

1. Phthalates are found in dish soap, air fresheners, and toilet paper, among other products. It's part of the products fragrance and so won't be listed as an ingredient. Phthalates are endocrine disruptors. In men, higher phthalate levels correspond to reduce sperm count.

2. Perchloroethylene or *perc* is found in spot removers, dry-cleaning solutions, and upholstery

and carpet cleaners. It's classified by the EPA as a possible carcinogen. Side effects from exposure are loss of coordination and dizziness, among others.

3. Triclosan is most commonly found in so-called *antibacterial* hand soaps and liquid dishwashing detergents. Triclosan is a possible carcinogen and its runoff has proven dangerous to algae.

4. Quarternary Ammonium Compounds, or *quats*, are found in antibacterial household cleaners and fabric softer liquids and dryer sheets. Quats are skin irritants and may have links to asthma and other respiratory disorders.

5. 2-Butoxyethanol is found in multipurpose cleaners, as well as kitchen and window cleaners. It's been linked to sore throats, pulmonary edema (caused by excess fluid in the lungs), narcosis, severe kidney and liver damage.

6. Ammonia is found in metal and porcelain polishing agents, and glass cleaners. It may have an immediate detrimental effect on those who suffer from lung issues, asthma, bronchitis, or other

breathing problems. It can also interact dangerously with bleach, creating a poisonous gas much like chloroform.

7. Chlorine is found in toilet bowl cleaners, laundry whiteners, mildew removers, toilet bowl cleaners, and household tap water. Chlorine is a thyroid disrupter.

8. Sodium Hydroxide is often found in drain openers and oven cleaners. It can be extremely corrosive to skin and eyes, nose and throat.

But here are some healthier cleaning alternatives for the home!

- Choose fragrance-free or all-natural organic products
- Skip air fresheners, open a window
- Take dry-clean clothes, sheets and drapes to a wet cleaner, find one online
- Buy cleansers using liquid carbon dioxide (CO_2)
- Avoid antibacterial cleaners
- Use alcohol-based hand sanitizers without triclosan

- Use vinegar as a natural fabric softener
- Use antifungal, antibacterial tea-tree oil (mixed with vinegar and lavender for scent) as an all-purpose cleaner
- Clean windows and mirrors with diluted vinegar and newspaper
- Use Bon Ami powder as an alternative to commercial cleansers
- Use vodka to polish metal or mirrors
- Use toothpaste as a silver polish
- Use baking soda and vinegar to clear clogged drains

Natural soaps and body care products have the same benefits. Industrial makeups, deodorants, shampoos, moisturizers, and shampoos often contain questionable chemicals such as:

1. Parabens: Chemicals such as propylparabens, methylparabens, ethylparabens, and butylparabens, which preserve shelf-life. Parabens are commonly found in makeup, body wash, night cream, face wash, shampoo. They mimic estrogen and create hormonal imbalance. Parabens are also

closely associated with breast cancer and fertility/reproductive issues.

2. Phthalates increase flexibility in cosmetics. They're commonly found in deodorants, lotions, and hair spray. Phthalates are endocrine disrupters and may cause birth defects.

3. Fragrance is a collection of dangerous chemicals and is most often found in hand creams, moisturizers, and hair products. It can cause allergies, reproductive issues, infertility, and hormone disruption.

4. Sodium Laureth Sulfate (SLES) and/or Sodium Lauryl Sulfate (SLS) are found in body wash, shampoo, and bubble bath. They can trigger allergies and cause skin irritation.

5. BHT are synthetic antioxidants which extend shelf life. They're most commonly found in lipstick, diaper creams, moisturizers. BHT are likely carcinogens, hormone disrupters, and may cause severe live damage.

6. Retinyl palmitate and Retinol (aka, Vitamin A) found in anti-aging skincare creams and

moisturizers. It may speed skin tumor growth and damage DNA.

7. Lead is a neurotoxin and heavy metal found in lipstick, lip gloss, and Vaseline. Lead is closely tied to learning and behavioral problems.

8. Formaldehyde is commonly used in most cosmetics. It's a known carcinogen and is closely linked to neurotoxicity, asthma, and developmental toxicity.

A new natural retinol alternative, bakuchiol, has come out and has incredible anti-aging benefits. It gives you similar results to retinol without the irritation. This is the skincare line I've been using while pregnant and my skin has never looked better—never thought I'd say that while pregnant!

Here are some healthy alternatives to the dangerous cosmetics and soaps. Take note that these are specific brands and we as publishers have no association with them, privately or publicly. This is not a commercial endorsement, and we recommend you research all these products thoroughly as part of your own due diligence:

- Pure Deodorant
- Citrus Mimosa Body Butter
- Volume & Shape Mist
- Adaptive Moisture Lotion
- Citrus Rosemary Body Oil
- Hydrating Body Lotion
- Citrus Mimosa Hand Cream
- Sea Salt Spray
- Daily Shampoo
- Citrus Mimosa Body Wash
- Kid's Body Wash
- Baby All-Over Wash
- Sheer Lipstick
- Nourishing Day Cream
- Calming Diaper Rash Cream
- Dew Skin Tinted Moisturizer
- Antioxidant Soft Cream (Day Cream)
- Tripeptide Radiance Serum
- Overnight Resurfacing Peel
- Tetrapeptide Supreme Cream
- Ultra Renewal Eye Cream

- Sheer Lipstick
- Sheer Lip Gloss
- Color Intense Lipstick

That's another big boatload of information, we're well aware. But don't be daunted. Remember that this book is a much a reference book as anything else, designed to be re-read and reviewed as needed.

However, it should hardly be surprising, with fasting and cleansing and other related practices becoming more popular, that cleansing/detox kits would be made available, virtual one-stop-shops for at-home treatment. Without any endorsement, let's look at some of the leading and easy ways to pursue cleansing your body of toxins.

CHAPTER NINE:
Popular Cleanses

It's easy enough to use water for a cleanse, but there are also cleansing kits made available from different producers for different purposes. So let's take a look at some of the popular cleanses which are prepacked to give you the maximum nutritional value and impact. Remember that we're not associated with any of these producers. We're here for you, not for them. But one or more might just be perfect for your needs. We're here to give you choices, to give you information. Use it well! Always consult with your doctor before changing your dietary or exercise protocols!

Juice Cleanses

Juice cleanses are popular, varied, and controversial. Some are steadfast supporters and a lot of detractors. Holistic nutritionists support the idea that juices cleanses help the body to take a break from the heavy foods and potentially allergenic foods in favor of easily digested and assimilated nutrients of pure vegetables and fruits. The juices detoxify and hydrate at the same time, a clear plus.

Raw Generation has the standard juice cleanses, the company also offers a signature Protein Cleanse. Available in three-, five-, and seven-day options, the cleanse proports to cleanse the body without sacrificing the adequate consumption of protein or the energy which goes along with it. The options sell for between $100 and $250 or so and contain six juices and 40 grams of plant protein.

Pressed Juicery has been a respected name in juice cleansing for years. They offer an extensive menu of over 20 juice blends and cleanse packages in three bundles. Their beginner cleanse, most popular cleanse, and experienced bundles all sell for about $30 dollars.

The company Suja offers a signature 3-Day Juice Cleanse for about $100, which features healthy breakfast recipes and a seven-juice cleanse.

Juice Generation is the purveyor of Citrus Super C, a delicious and well-missed beverage. They currently offer thee Cooler Cleanses, in one-, three-, and five-day packages costing from roughly $60 to roughly $300. These cleanses focus on the juices, unlike Suja. Their Blend It Yourself offering, the ingredients are delivered to you to mix at home, reducing plastic consumption and lowering your carbon footprint.

Juiced offers an affordable and convenient juice cleanse which is designed to jumpstart and energize healthier lifestyle habits. Introducing blended, raw veggies and fruits into the user's daily routine for as long as a full week, their Jumpstart Cleanse costs less than $30 a day. This cleanse proports to improve response to stress, break the sugar-craving cycle, boost focus and mental clarity, and more. This regiment offers seven juice drinks a day, plus unlimited raw fruits and vegetables.

Project Juice' has organic juice cleanses which include three different five-day options, plus the user has the option to create a custom regiment.

The company offers a beginners-level Classic Reset Cleanse and an experienced-level Advanced Reset Cleanse. Each costs about $75 per day and includes six juice drinks a day. The company's premium package is their Immunity Reboot Cleanse includes two very potent wellness shots every day at roughly $85 per day.

Lemonkind has a 3-Day Reset Core Juice Cleanse which features 24 juices (eight per day for three days). The cleanse is designed to break bad habits, detox the body, jumpstart a healthier diet. The regiment calls for a hearty juice drink every two hours, which makes it more satisfying and easier to follow.

Squeezed is an excellent choice for those unwilling to commit. The company offers various options to ease the user's transition into the cleanse. They have programs that go from one day to seven, at roughly $30 per day. Raw vegetables and fruits are permitted during the week.

Three Cleanses to Avoid

Not everybody agrees about the all-juice cleanse. People have tried it and recorded their experiences online and they are often anything but glowing. A diet of warm lemon water and several bottles of juice may provide less than 1000 calories, leaving a lot of people feeling hungry, irritable, and weak. This can also lead to headaches and a distinct lack of sociability. Many experts believe that juices the fruits rob them of the fiber and nutrients the whole fruits offer.

The tea cleanse also has its detractors. Stomach cramps and sleep deprivation are often reported with these cleanse types. Tea is also a laxative, so it may evacuate residual feces and water, but it won't change the fat-to-muscle ratio.

Drinking tea can have a lot of positive effects, but being a full-body cleanser simply isn't one of them.

There's a cleanse known as The Master Cleanse, but it makes some outrageous claims.

According to the purveyors of this plan, the human body can survive off nothing more than six to 12 glasses of a concoction made of maple syrup, lemon juice, cayenne pepper, and water, for up to ten days. The claim is that up to 20 pounds can be lost in those ten days. The Master Cleanse seeks to help users overcome a psychological need to eat. And while there are connections between psychology and eating disorders, there are physiological needs to eat which have to be addressed. Ten days is longer than almost any expert will recommend going without eating.

Dedicated Cleansing Kits

A product called zuPOO proports to be able to flush out between five and 20 pounds of fecal matter from the bowel. This is important for the body, as we've seen, one of the many reasons for a colon cleanse. It's important to remember that fasts and cleanses in general achieve this same thing. Whether zuPOO is more effective than more DIY cleanses will be for the user to decide. It certainly should deliver a smoother digestion once the bowels are cleared, in any case.

The company offers a powerful blend of minerals, vitamins, herbs, and barks which it claims flush waste matter out of the system. This evacuation is said to begin with one to two days of administration, and the product is recommended for use in a 15-day cycle to fully flush out the bowels. (Keep in mind this includes good bacteria as well as bad.) The formula includes six natural ingredients with special functionality:

Cascara Sagrada, a gentle, natural laxative, is proven effective against constipation, a potent boost to the immune system, and a good way to promote probiotic bacteria.

Bentonite clay draws waste out of the body and passes it. The clay includes magnesium, calcium, sodium, silica, iron, copper, and potassium, all beneficial minerals.

Aloe ferox is well-known for its colon-cleansing powers. A 2004 study found that 30% of participants using the aloe demonstrated improvement or clinical remission. Only one percent of participants who took a placebo presented the same results.

Milk thistle is known to be a powerful fortifier of the liver, supporting liver function and tissue health.

Cayenne pepper, which we've already looked at briefly, has been shown to have a very positive effect on the human digestive system. It encourages saliva production, important for good digestion and fighting bad breath. Cayenne pepper is also known to stimulate enzyme production, essential for proper digestive system functionality. Cayenne pepper is also proven to stimulate gastric juices which aid the human body's metabolism of food and toxins.

Slippery Elm Extract has demonstrated a 20% increase in frequency of bowel movement frequency. Users have also reported less abdominal pain, bloating, and straining, and improvements in the consistency of stool. It can improve digestion and aid in weight loss.

It's taken in capsules, one or two in the evening before bed. Gas may build up in the first day or two. Flushing should begin after 12 hours or so.

Tips for Cleansing

Fiber is important. Eat enough brown rice, organic fresh vegetables and fruits, including:
- Beets
- Radishes
- Artichokes
- Cabbage
- Broccoli
- Spirulina
- Chlorella
- Seaweed

Protect and cleanse the liver with herbs such as:
- Burlock
- Dandelion root

- Milk thistle
- Green tea
- Vitamin C
- Glutathione

Experts recommend:

- Drinking two quarts of water per day or more
- Deep breathing for oxygenation of the system
- Emphasizing positive emotions to transform stress
- Hydrotherapy, in the form of a hot five-minute shower followed by 30 seconds of cold water (do this three times in a row and go to bed for at least 30 minutes)
- Saunas to encourage sweating to eliminate waste
- Dry-brush skin or use foot spas/baths which remove toxins through the pores of the skin.

And that's about it for cleanses. And once your body is cleansed, it's time to move on to picking the right diet. Because cleansing and fasting may help you lose weight, but it won't keep the weight off and it likely will not get off all the weight you want to lose. These are ways of kickstarting your new lifestyle, but a good diet is the way to make it a reality. So let's move on to the subject of perhaps more self-help books than any other.

Dieting.

SECTION 4: DIETING

CHAPTER TEN:
Ketogenic Diet

Think back to the ugly statistics about obesity and ill-health. You already know the importance of a good diet by now, and you likely had some idea before picking up this book. But a good diet is both effective for weight loss and for weight management, and some are particularly good for an intermittent fasting lifestyle.

Keep in mind that fasting itself is a kind of diet, a crash diet of only water, minimal caloric intake, etc. But a diet is a regiment, and one of the most popular regiments these days in the ketogenic diet.

We looked at the ketogenic diet briefly. To remind you, the body generally uses carbohydrates as a preferred source of fuel, allowing fat to collect. Denying the body carbohydrates leaves the body to use its resources of energy from carbs and turns to using fats for fuel. Once the body goes through ketosis and reprograms itself to use fat as the preferred source of fuel, creating brain-feeding ketones, fat stores are used and no longer collect so readily. The ketogenic diet lowers levels of insulin too, and that is beneficial for boosting blood sugar management and insulin sensitivity.

The ketogenic diet has a high fat content, moderate protein content, and low carbohydrate content. It only takes a few weeks for the shift to occur.

Ketogenic staple foods include:

- Meat
- Butter
- Cheese
- Fish
- Eggs
- Heavy cream
- Nuts
- Oils
- Seeds
- Avocados
- Low-carb vegetables

It's probably no surprise that a lot of those foods seem familiar, especially from the cleanses and post-fasting foods. This is what makes the ketogenic such a good diet for before or after fasting. The ketogenic diet eliminates nearly all (and also familiar) sources of carbohydrates, including:

- Rice
- Grains
- Potatoes
- Beans
- Milk
- Sugars
- Fruits
- Cereals
- High-carb veggies

Does it work? The ketogenic diet has been shown to lower insulin levels, increase fat burning, and producing brain-nourishing ketones. It may create fat loss, muscle gain, and improve disease markers. Some studies suggest that, given the same calorie intake, a ketogenic diet can be more effective for weight loss than a low-fat diet. One study produced a similar results: volunteers on the ketogenic diet lost over two times more weight than volunteers on a low-fat, low-calorie diet. HDL (high density, or good) cholesterol, and triglyceride levels also increased. Calories in both groups were reduced equally.

A 2007 study compared a low-carb regiment to the dietary guidelines of Diabetes UK. dietary guidelines. The low-fat group lost 4.6 pounds (2.1 kg). The low-carb group lost 15.2 pounds (6.9 kg). Over 3 months, the low-carb diet generated three times more weight loss over three months.

Specialists aren't certain as to whether these results are from a metabolic advantage to the ketogenic diets or simply higher protein intake. There's also some question about long-term results from the ketogenic diet.

The ketogenic diet works through a series of processes to promote weight loss:

- Higher protein intake, which has many weight-loss benefits

- Gluconeogenesis, converting fat and protein into carbohydrates for fuel, burning calories
- Appetite suppressant, supported by changes in leptin and ghrelin and other hunger hormones
- Improved insulin sensitivity, improving metabolism and fuel utilization
- Decreased fat storage by reducing lipogenesis, the process of converting sugar into fat
- Increased fat burning

Ketogenic Diet and Metabolic Diseases

We took a brief look at metabolic syndrome, common risk factors for type 2 diabetes like obesity, and heart disease. Others include:
- High blood pressure
- High waist-to-hip ratio (excess belly fat)
- High levels of LDL (bad) cholesterol
- Low levels of HDL (good) cholesterol
- High blood sugar levels

Many of these risk factors may be improved or eliminated with some lifestyle and nutritional changes.

Insulin plays a big role in metabolic diseases and diabetes in particular. Ketogenic diets are known to lower insulin levels, particularly for sufferers of prediabetes or type 2 diabetes. One study revealed that after two weeks of being on a ketogenic diet, insulin sensitivity was improved by 75% while blood sugar dropped considerably, from a high of 7.5 mmol/l to a low of 6.2 mmol/l. Another study revealed a 16% blood sugar reduction. Seven out of 21 volunteers stopped using diabetic medication after the study. Other studies in animals and humans found the ketogenic diet reducing total triglycerides and cholesterol levels.

It's important to note that some studies found negative effects of the ketogenic diet in children. Also, research indicates that saturated fat intake as happens in the ketogenic diet may increase levels of LDL (low-density, or bad) cholesterol, a big risk factor for heart disease. Other studies demonstrate a connection between cancer and some fats.

Impact of the Ketogenic Diet on Metabolic Disease

Key factors of the ketogenic diet effect certain markers of metabolic disease, including:
- Fewer carbs: High carbs mean higher insulin and blood sugar, decreasing insulin resistance
- Decreased insulin resistance: This causes high trigiyceride levels, inflammation, and fat storage
- Ketone bodies: These protect against cancer, epilepsy, Alzheimer's, and other diseases
- Reduced inflammation: The ketogenic diet reduces inflammation, linked to metabolic syndrome
- Fat loss: Abdominal fat, a staple of metabolic disease, is vulnerable to the ketogenic diet

- Restoration of insulin function: Healthy insulin levels fight inflammation

Is the Ketogenic Diet Right for You?

Diets vary, as do people. No diet is perfect for everyone. The right diet depends on a variety of factors, including lifestyle, heredity, tastes, and so on. The ketogenic diet is also not suitable for sufferers of:
- Liver failure
- Pancreatitis
- Carnitine deficiency
- Fat metabolism disorders
- Pyruvate kinase deficiency
- Porphyrias

Dieters should also be wary of the so-called *keto flu*, a collection of flu-like symptoms including:
- Low energy
- Digestive discomfort
- Nausea
- Poor exercise performance

- Poor mental function
- Increased hunger
- Sleep issues
- Dehydration

There may also be risks to liver and kidneys after extended periods on the ketogenic diet, though the research is lacking in this department.

A ketogenic diet isn't always easy to stick to. Carb cycling or a low-carbohydrate diet may be preferable. Athletes may find the use of fat inconvenient, as they rely more on carbs, and vegans and vegetarians may balk at the reliance on meats and dairy.

As we've seen changing the body's energy source from carbohydrates to fat can increase ketones in the blood. This so-called *dietary ketosis* is different from *ketoacidosis,* a very dangerous condition.

Too many ketones may cause ketoacidosis (DKA). DKA is prevalent in type 1 diabetes, where excessive blood glucose can occur from lack of insulin. It's also possible in type 2 diabetes when ketone levels get too high. Being on a low-carb diet like the ketogenic diet while ill may increase the risk of DKA. DKA is considered a medical emergency. Symptoms require immediate medical attention, as the sufferer may fall into a diabetic coma.

DKA warning signs include:
- Dry mouth
- Consistently high blood sugar
- Nausea
- Frequent urination
- Breathing difficulties
- Fruit-like odor in the breath

We've already taken a look at the keto-friendly foods, but let's be a bit more specific, as we're about to move on to an entire keto-friendly menu!

A ketogenic diet should center around these foods:
- Eggs: Organic, pasteurized whole eggs are best
- Poultry: Turkey or chicken only
- Shellfish: Oysters, shrimp and scallops

- Fatty fish: Herring, mackerel, wild salmon
- Meat: Venison, bison, pork, venison, grass-fed beef, organ meats
- Full-fat dairy: Butter, yogurt, and cream.
- Full-fat cheese: Mozzarella, cheddar, brie, cream cheese, goat cheese
- Nuts and seeds: Almonds, macadamia nuts, walnuts, peanuts pumpkin seeds and flaxseeds
- Nut butter: Natural almond, peanut, and cashew butters
- Healthy fats: Olive oil, coconut oil, avocado oil, sesame oil, coconut butter
- Avocado: Whole avocados
- Non-starchy vegetables: Broccoli, greens, mushrooms, tomatoes, peppers
- Condiments: Pepper, salt, lemon juice, fresh herbs, spices. vinegar

  Keto-friendly beverage choices include:
- Water: The best source of hydration
- Sparkling water: A good replacement for soda

- Unsweetened coffee: Flavored with heavy cream instead of sugar
- Unsweetened green tea: Especially green tea

The following foods should be restricted:

- Breads and baked goods: Breads, cookies, crackers, rolls, and doughnuts
- Sweet, sugary foods: Ice cream, sugar, maple syrup. candy, maple syrup, coconut
- Sweetened drinks: Juices, soda, sports drinks, flavored teas
- Pasta: All forms of noodles
- Grain products: Rice, wheat, cereals, oats, tortillas
- Starchy vegetables: Butternut squash, potatoes, corn, sweet potatoes, pumpkin, peas
- Beans and legumes: Chickpeas, black beans, kidney beams, lentils
- Fruit: Grapes, citrus, pineapple, bananas
- Sauces: sweet salad dressing, barbecue sauce, dipping sauces

- Some alcoholic beverages: Sugary mixed drinks, beer
- Unhealthy fats: margarine, vegetable oils like corn and canola, shortening
- Processed foods: Packaged foods, fast foods, and processed meats
- Diet foods: Preservatives, artificial colors, sweeteners like aspartame and sugar alcohols

A One-Week Sample Keto Menu

Note: The recipes which follow are all based on reasonable portions. While proportions of one ingredient over another depend on taste, we're basing these meals on a few standard measurements which should be applied across the board. Salad recipes are based on two cups of greens. Limit salad dressings to two tablespoons. Cream cheese or nut butters should be limited to one tablespoon. Cheese portions should be limited to two slices or one ounce. Vegetable and fruit portions between one and five pieces, depending on the size. Meat portions are generally six to eight ounces. All diets recommend six to eight glasses of water each day.

This menu was put together by dietary experts. It offers fewer than 50 grams of carbohydrates per day.

Monday

- Breakfast: Two fried eggs (pastured butter only) with sauteed greens
- Lunch: Grass-fed burger patty (no bun) topped with mushrooms cheese, and avocado on a bed of greens
- Dinner: Pork chops, sauteed green beans (coconut oil)

Tuesday

- Breakfast: Mushroom and cheese omelet
- Lunch: Tuna salad (with celery), a slice of beefsteak tomato, served on a bed of greens.
- Dinner: Roast chicken topped with cream sauce and served with sauteed broccoli (pasteurized butter)

Wednesday
- Breakfast: Stuffed bell pepper (cheese and eggs)
- Lunch: Arugula salad topped with turkey, blue cheese, hard-boiled eggs, and avocado
- Dinner: Grilled wild-caught salmon served with sauteed spinach (coconut oil)

Thursday
- Breakfast: Yogurt (full-fat) with Keto granola and/or blueberries
- Lunch: Steak bowl (cauliflower rice, herbs, cheese, salsa, avocado)
- Dinner: Bison steak with broccoli in a cheese sauce

Friday
- Breakfast: Baked avocado and eggs (whole)
- Lunch: Caesar salad with grilled chicken
- Dinner: Roasted or grilled pork chops with apple sauce and roasted vegetables

Saturday
- Breakfast: Cauliflower toast with avocado, cheese, and ground pepper

- Lunch: Wild-caught salmon burgers drizzled with pesto
- Dinner: Zucchini noodles and meatballs with parmesan cheese

Sunday

- Breakfast: Coconut milk chia pudding topped with walnuts and coconut
- Lunch: Cobb salad (greens, avocado, hard-boiled eggs, turkey, cheese)
- Dinner: Coconut chicken curry with cauliflower rice.

That's a week of satisfying and keto-friendly meals. But everybody likes to snack every now and then. So here are some healthy ketogenic snacks:

- Cheddar cheese and almonds
- An avocado half stuffed with homemade chicken salad
- Low-carb vegetables with guacamole
- Unsweetened trail mix
- Cocoanut chips
- Hard-boiled eggs
- Sliced salami and olives (green or black)

- Kale chips
- Peppers and celery with cream cheese dip
- Berries topped with heavy whipping cream
- Beef jerky
- Greens with avocado and high-fat dressing
- Macadamia nuts
- Avocado cocoa mousse
- Keto smoothie made with coconut milk, cocoa and avocado

The Ketogenic diet certainly has gotten a lot of attention, and that is only fitting. You'll note how elements of this diet recur in other popular diets. And there are other popular diets, after all. Let's take a closer look at them now.

CHAPTER ELEVEN:
Other Popular Diets

The Paleo Diet

The paleo diet (also called the paleolithic or the *stone age* diet) is based on foods which are similar to those available during the paleolithic era, which lasted between 2.5 million to (as recently as) 10,000 years ago. This includes fish, lean meats, vegetables, fruits, seeds and nuts. Since farming became popular about 10,000 years ago, at the end of the paleolithic era, dairy products, grains, and legumes are also included (unlike the ketogenic diet).

The reasoning behind the paleo diet is that the body's genetic makeup does not fit its modern, processed diet. It holds that our bodies are basically unchanged from the paleolithic era, though our environment has changed drastically, as we've already discussed. This is called the *discordance hypothesis*.

People who choose the paleo diet often have similar goals, and a full body detox is often one of them. You may want to lose weight or to maintain an optimal and healthy body weight. Others may want assistance in meal-planning.

Like the ketogenic diet, the paleo diet comes with some variation, which makes it more flexible. In general, a new paleo dieter will be looking forward to eating the following foods:

- Fruits
- Vegetables
- Fruits
- Lean meats (grass-fed or wild game)
- Nuts and seeds
- Fish (salmon, albacore tuna, mackerel, any that are rich in omega-3 fatty acids
- Olive oil or walnut oil
  The paleo diet basically avoids these foods:
- Grains: Wheat, barley, and oats

- Legumes: Lentils, beans, peas, peanuts
- Salt
- Dairy products
- Potatoes
- Refined sugar
- Processed foods

A Typical Paleo Diet Daily Menu

Just a reminder: These following recipes also follow reasonable-portion measurements. Salad recipes are based on two cups of greens. Limit salad dressings to two tablespoons. Cream cheese or nut butters should be limited to one tablespoon. Cheese portions should be limited to two slices or one ounce. Vegetable and fruit portions between one and five pieces, depending on the size. Meat portions are generally six to eight ounces. All diets recommend six to eight glasses of water each day.

With that in mind, here's a look at the first of several different sample menus, this one delineating what you might eat during a typical day following a paleo diet:

- Breakfast: Broiled salmon served with cantaloupe.
- Lunch: Broiled pork loin served with a salad (romaine, cucumber, carrot, walnut, tomatoes, tossed with lemon juice dressing).
- Dinner: Beef sirloin tri-tip (roast), steamed spinach or broccoli, salad (mixed greens, avocado, tomatoes, onions, topped with almonds and tossed with lemon juice dressing), and strawberries for dessert.
- Snacks: Celery stalks, carrot sticks, an orange.

A One Week's Sample Paleo Menu

Monday

- Breakfast: Kale, avocado, apple, banana, and almond milk smoothie

- Lunch: Mixed salad with fried seabass and pumpkin seeds, tossed in an olive oil dressing
- Dinner: Roast chicken with stuffing (carrots, onions, rosemary)

Tuesday

- Breakfast: Scrambled eggs with grilled tomatoes, spinach, and pumpkin seeds
- Lunch: Mixed salad with roast chicken, tossed in an olive oil dressing
- Dinner: Baked salmon with broccoli and asparagus (fried in coconut oil)

Wednesday

- Breakfast: Chopped bananas with almonds and blueberries
- Lunch: Mixed salad with salmon and tossed with an olive oil dressing
- Dinner: Stir-fry beef with onions and mixed peppers (fried in coconut oil)

Thursday

- Breakfast: Coconut oil-fried broccoli with a poached egg and toasted almonds

- Lunch: Mixed salad with boiled eggs, tuna, olive oil, and sesame seeds
- Dinner: Harissa-baked chicken legs or wings, served with steamed broccoli

Friday

- Breakfast: Spinach, mixed berries, and coconut milk smoothie
- Lunch: Broccoli, tomato, and butternut squash omelet, served with a mixed salad
- Dinner: Salmon stir-fry with broccoli, red pepper, baby corn

Saturday

- Breakfast: Eggs, bacon, and tomatoes pan-fried in virgin olive oil
- Lunch: Chicken and vegetable soup, served with turmeric
- Dinner: Lamb chops (grilled or roasted) with spiced red cabbage and spinach

Sunday

- Breakfast: Mushroom, tomato, and spring onion omelet

- Lunch: Mixed salad with avocado, chicken, olive oil, seeds
- Dinner: Beef stew and mixed vegetables.

Between meals, drinking water and getting plenty of exercise is recommended. The diet also emphasizes drinking water and being physically active every day. Several clinical trials compared the paleo diet to the Mediterranean Diet and the Diabetes Diet. They showed that the paleo diet may provide special benefits, including:

- Greater weight loss
- Improved blood pressure levels
- Greater glucose tolerance
- Better appetite management
- Lower triglycerides

The Mediterranean Diet

The Mediterranean diet is popular among doctors and nutritionists for the prevention of disease and maintain better health for longer. The Mediterranean diet is inspired by the foods of the countries surrounding the Mediterranean Sea, including Italy, Greece, and France. The diet emphasizes these foods:

- Fish
- Healthful fats
- Legumes
- Nuts
- Olive oil
- Vegetables
- Fruits
- Vegetables
- Whole grains
- Red wine
- Purple grapes
- Dark chocolate

The diet de-emphasizes these foods:

- Dairy
- Eggs
- Meat
- Refined grains (white flour)
- Refined oils (including soybean and canola oils)

- Sugary foods (pastries, sodas)
- Processed meats (hot dogs, deli meats)
- Packaged or processed foods

Like the ketogenic diet, the Mediterranean diet has a higher percentage of calories from fat than other diet regiments. Those are monounsaturated fats (like olive oil) so it may not be right for people watching their fat intake.

A One Week's Sample Mediterranean Menu

Note: With every day, a breakfast option of Greek yogurt with walnuts and blueberries is allowed.

Monday

- Breakfast: one fried egg on whole-wheat toast with grilled tomatoes and sliced avocado
- Lunch: Mixed salad greens with cherry tomatoes and olives on top and a dressing of olive oil and vinegar whole-grain pita bread 2 ounces (oz) of hummus

- Dinner: Whole-grain crust pizza with tomato sauce, various grilled low-carb vegetables, low-fat cheese, small pieces of ham, or chicken.

Tuesday

- Breakfast:1 cup of Greek yogurt with half a cup of fruits, such as blueberries, raspberries, or chopped nectarines. For additional calories, add 1–2 oz of almonds or walnuts.
- Lunch: Whole-grain bread sandwich with grilled vegetables (zucchini, eggplant, union, bell pepper) and spread with hummus or avocado.
- Dinner: Baked salmon or cod with black pepper and garlic, one roasted potato drizzled in olive oil and sprinkled with chives

Wednesday

- Breakfast: Whole-grain oats with dates, cinnamon, and honey topped with low-sugar fruits (blackberries or raspberries) shredded almonds (these are optional)

- Lunch: Boiled white beans with garlic, laurel, and cumin. Raw arugula tossed in an olive oil dressing and topped with cucumber, tomato, and feta cheese
- Dinner: Whole-grain pasta with olive oil, tomato sauce, grilled vegetables, Parmesan cheese

Thursday

- Breakfast: Two scrambled eggs (with onions, bell peppers, tomatoes topped with queso fresco
- Lunch: Roasted anchovies on whole-grain toast with lemon juice, served with a warm salad of steamed tomatoes and kale
- Dinner: Steamed spinach with herbs and lemon juice, a boiled artichoke with salt, garlic powder, and olive oil.

Friday

- Breakfast: Greek yogurt with honey and cinnamon, shredded almonds and chopped apple

- Lunch: Quinoa with sun-dried tomatoes, bell peppers, roasted garbanzo beans (with thyme and oregano), olives, topped with avocado or feta cheese crumbles
- Dinner: Steamed kale with cucumber, tomato, lemon juice, olives, and Parmesan cheese, grilled sardines served with a slice of lemon

Saturday

- Breakfast: Whole-grain toast (two slices) with soft cheese (queso fresco, ricotta, or goat) add chopped blueberries or figs
- Lunch: Mixed greens with cucumber and tomato, roasted chicken, olive oil, lemon juice
- Dinner: Vegetables roasted in olive oil (carrot, artichoke, eggplant, zucchini, tomato, sweet potato), served with one cup of whole-grain couscous

Sunday

- Breakfast: whole-grain oats with dates, cinnamon, maple syrup, low-sugar fruits

- Lunch: stewed yellow squash, zucchini, potato, onion, topped with a tomato/herb sauce
- Dinner: Spinach or arugula with olives, olive oil, tomato, a portion of white fish

Suitable snacks include:

- A small portion of nuts
- Whole fruits (oranges, grapes, plums)
- Dried fruits (figs and apricots)
- A small portion of yogurt
- A small portion of hummus with carrots, celery, or other low-calorie vegetables
- Whole-grain toast with avocado

The Atkins Diet

The Atkins diet, like the ketogenic diet, promotes low-carb intake for weight loss, though it may also improve or prevent various health conditions, such as heart disease and high blood pressure.

The Atkins diet was first created in 1972, but it's evolved a lot since then. Today, fifty years later, there are two distinct Atkins diets. Atkins 20 is the original diet, described below and based on a net carb intake of only 20 grams. The new Atkins 40 is not as and allows 40 grams of net carbs, double that of the first regiment.

Both versions of the diet consist of proteins, healthy fats, and vegetables (comparable to the ketogenic diet). In fact, some people consider the Atkins diet as a precursor to the ketogenic diet.

The Atkins diet features a Food Guide Pyramid, prioritizing food from bottom (to be eaten more) to top (to be eaten less). The pyramid includes whole grains such as oats, rice, and barley.

The pyramid does not include so-called *white foods*, including:
- White rice
- White sugar
- White potatoes
- White bread

- Pasta made with white flour

The Atkins diet is constructed and applied in phases. Net carbs vary in each phase.

Phase 1: Induction. This is where the regiment is the strictest. Dieters must forgo, entirely:

- Bread
- Fruit
- Starchy vegetables
- Grains
- Alcohol
- Dairy products (other than butter and cheese)

Phase 1 allows 20 grams of net carbs per day. The FDA recommends 300 grams daily. The idea is to increase the body's fat-burning ability. It's effective and motivational.

Phase 2 is notable for ongoing weight loss even as a few whole food carbs are reintroduced to the diet. These include:

- Legumes
- Berries
- Tomato juice

- Nuts
- Yogurt

Phase 2 allows 25 to 50 net carbohydrates per day. Phase 2 goes on until the dieter is within roughly 10 pounds of their target weight.

Phase 3 focuses on pre-maintenance and continues to add a increasing variety of carbohydrates, including more fruits, whole grains, and starchy vegetables.

Phase 3 allows between 50 to 80 net carbohydrates per day. This phase continues for roughly a month after reaching target weight.

Phase 4 is lifetime maintenance employing a low-carbohydrate (80-100 net carbohydrates daily) diet for the rest of the dieter's life.

If all this sounds familiar, it's because the Atkins diet relies on the same process of ketosis which the ketogenic diet uses.

A Journal of the American Medical Association study found that women on the Atkins diet lost 10 pounds on average and showed lower blood pressure and improved triglyceride levels.

But the Atkins diet suffers from the same drawback as the ketogenic diet; high fat intake is a danger to liver, kidneys, heart, and other organs and various systems throughout the body. Potassium and vitamin C are notably missing from the Atkins diet as well.

A One Week's Sample Atkins Menu

Like the current ketogenic diet (and really, Atkins is a ketogenic diet at heart), the Atkins diet is made up of 60–70% fat, 20–30% protein, and five to ten percent carbs. Net carb intake is limited to between 20 and 40 grams daily, mostly from mineral- and vitamin-rich vegetables. This sample diet averages about 20.5g daily net carbs.

Monday
- Breakfast: Scrambled eggs with cheddar cheese and sautéed onions

- Lunch: Deli ham over mixed greens with avocado, 5 large black olives, sliced cucumbers, and blue cheese dressing
- Dinner: Baked Catfish served with broccoli and butter
- Snacks: Atkins Peanut Butter Fudge Crisp Bar, 3/4 sliced zucchini and provolone cheese

Tuesday

- Breakfast: Atkins Frozen Sausage Scramble
- Lunch: Tuna salad with mixed greens, 3 cherry tomatoes
- Dinner: Lean pork chop served with cauliflower and cheddar cheese
- Snacks: Sliced red bell pepper with ranch dressing, celery with cream cheese

Wednesday

- Breakfast: Swiss cheese and spinach omelet
- Lunch: Grilled chicken over baby spinach, tomato, and avocado salad
- Dinner: Sauteed beef and vegetables over a bed of romaine

- Snacks: Atkins strawberry shake, ham with cream cheese, and a dill pickle spear

Thursday

- Breakfast: Spinach and cheese omelet with avocado and salsa on top
- Lunch: Atkins frozen crustless chicken pot pie
- Dinner: Hamburger topped with pepper jack cheese, small tomato, avocado, and romaine lettuce
- Snacks: Atkins French vanilla shake, Zucchini and Monterey jack cheese

Friday

- Breakfast: Two eggs, shredded cheddar cheese, salsa cruda
- Lunch: Atkins frozen chili con carne served with mixed greens and Italian dressing
- Dinner: Half of a cobb salad with ranch dressing
- Snacks: Atkins cafe caramel shake, sliced red bell pepper with ranch dressing

Saturday
- Breakfast: Red bell pepper stuffed with eggs scrambled with spinach and onion
- Lunch: Tuna salad (celery, dill pickle spear, mayonnaise)
- Dinner: Italian sausage, sliced onion and red bell pepper, served with baby spinach, sliced mushrooms, and blue cheese dressing
- Snacks: Atkins strawberry shake, one portobello mushroom cap stuffed with salsa cruda, and pepper jack cheese

Sunday
- Breakfast: Pumpkin pancakes
- Lunch: Grilled chicken breast served over romaine hearts with radishes and creamy Italian dressing
- Dinner: Baked Salmon served with charmoula and broccoli
- Snacks: Whole snap peas and cheddar cheese, celery and cream cheese

The Diabetes Diet

The diabetes diet is a plan for eating healthy that helps control blood sugar. Like a lot of the diets we've looked at so far (and all the best diets there are), the diabetes diet suggests eating only the healthiest food in moderate portions at regular mealtimes. The diet is rich in nutrients and low in calories and fat, relying heavily on whole grains, vegetables, and fruit. It's excellent diet for anyone on diabetes, naturally, but comes highly recommended for fasting, weight loss and weight management, and overall longevity. The diet may reduce risk of certain cancers and cardiovascular diseases. Consuming low-fat dairy products may reduce risk of low bone mass (osteoporosis loss of bone tissue).

Other benefits of the diabetes diet include:

- Control of blood sugar levels
- Control risk factors of heart disease and stroke
- Control high blood pressure

- Control high blood fats
- Prevent hyperglycemia, which can lead to kidney, nerve, and heart damage

The diet is great for these benefits, basically to control blood glucose levels, and weight loss.

The diabetes diet consists of three meals per day and always at regular times, which aids in insulin use. These meals focus on good fats, fish, fiber, and healthy carbohydrates.

Healthy carbohydrates? Sure! Carbs have their place, and not all carbs are the same. Sugars are simple carbohydrates, starches are complex carbohydrates which break down into blood glucose. So focus on healthy carbohydrates, such as:

- Vegetables
- Fruits
- Whole grains
- Legumes (peas and beans)
- Low-fat dairy (cheese and milk)

Fiber-rich foods include plant food and other things which the body doesn't absorb or digest and it helps moderate levels of blood sugar. High-fiber foods for this diet include:

- Fruits
- Vegetables
- Nuts
- Whole grains
- Legumes (peas and beans)

Heart-healthy fish are suggested for twice-weekly consumption. These include the fish we've looked at before (salmon, tuna, mackerel, sardines). Their wealth of omega-3 fatty acids may prevent various types of heart disease. Avoid frying the fish.

Just as there are healthy carbs, there are good fats, which we've already looked at in this book. These are the polyunsaturated and monounsaturated fats which lower cholesterol levels. Foods with these good fats include:

- Avocados
- Nuts
- Olive, peanut, and canola oils

Things to Avoid on the Diabetes Diet

Foods to avoid on the diabetes diet include any with saturated or trans fats. Saturated fats come from animal protein and high-fat dairy products. These include beef, butter, sausage, bacon, hot dogs, also palm kernel and cocoanut oils. Trans fats are found in baked goods, processed snacks, stick margarines, and shortening.

Avoid sources of cholesterol. They include organ meats, egg yolks, high-fat animal protein, and high-fat dairy products. The diabetes diet calls for 200 milligrams (mg) of cholesterol per day or less.

Avoid sodium. This diet calls for fewer than 2,300 mg daily. Sufferers of high blood pressure should consume even less.

Diabetes Diet Meal Plans

The American Diabetes Association has a simple and interesting way to balance meals on the diabetes diet. They call it the plate plan. It works by dividing your plate into quadrants for different foods: Half the plate is for non-starchy vegetables (carrots, spinach, tomatoes). One quarter of the plate with protein (lean pork, chicken, tuna) and the remaining quarter with a whole grain (rice) or starchy vegetable (green peas). Nuts and avocados may be added in small amounts. A serving of fruit or dairy may be added, and a glass of water or unsweetened coffee or tea.

A Sample Diabetes Diet Menu

This weekly menu provides 1,200 to 1,600 calories per day. It may be tailored for those who require more calories per day.

- Breakfast: Whole-wheat bread with jelly, shredded wheat cereal with one-percent percent low-fat milk, one piece of fruit, one cup of coffee
- Lunch: Roast beef sandwich (wheat bread, lettuce, tomato, low-fat American cheese, and mayonnaise) one apple, water
- Dinner: Salmon, small baked potato, carrots, green beans, one dinner roll, unsweetened iced tea (add milk to taste)
- Snack: Popcorn with margarine

The Hormone Diet

We've taken a look at how integral good hormonal balance is to overall good health, and how impactful hormonal imbalance can be. But hormones are complex; they're varied and diverse in form and function. For example, hormones can affect weight and can be affected by it. So whether a dieter is concerned about correcting hormonal imbalance or losing weight, both are likely to be affected by a change in diet.

It's well-known, for example, that hormonal fluctuations likely affect weight gain (particularly belly fat), sluggishness, lagging libido, stress, sugar cravings, and other health problems.

Some experts favor a variant on the Mediterranean diet, which proports to be good for weight loss and energy levels.

This approach, known as the glyci-med diet, starts with the Mediterranean diet but adds foods which are low on the glycemic index (these foods raise blood sugar slowly, whereas foods high on this index raise blood sugar quickly).

The hormone diet has proven beneficial for those suffering from diabetes, hypertension, and heart disease.

Like the Mediterranean diet, the best diet for hormone health includes:

- Lean protein (eggs, chicken breasts, wild-caught fish)

- Vegetables and most fruits (most nuts, flaxseeds, chia seeds, flaxseeds)
- Olive oil (unsaturated oils like canola)
- Whole grains (buckwheat, quinoa, brown rice)

  Meanwhile this minimizes or eliminates:
- Alcohol
- Caffeine
- Processed meats
- Fried foods
- Peanuts
- Full-fat dairy
- Saturated fat
- Artificial sweeteners
- Hi-GI carbohydrates

This diet does not indulge fasting. Dieters eat every three to four hours. The healthy meals will be consumed at a rate of 80%, leaving two meals out of ten as *cheat meals* to make the diet more sustainable. Some people observe the diet six days out of the week and give themselves a *cheat day*.

You'll eat often -- every 3-4 hours -- making healthy food choices at least 80% of the time. But you do get one to two "cheat meals" a week.

Like some of the other diets, the hormone diet is progressive. After a few weeks at the beginner level described above, dieters will advance to a medium-level regiment. It takes more effort, but it brings it better results. Note that it's best done progressively and it's not advised to jump into an advanced level without doing the beginning level first. This holds true for all the diets and regiments in this book.

For this next level, dieters abandon all alcohol, caffeine, diary, sugar, gluten, dairy, and most oils for at least two weeks. Instead, dieters add supplements, such as calcium, magnesium, vitamin D3, and omega-3 fatty acids.

As with all these diets (except the Atkins), the hormone diet relies on organic or whole foods, cooked fresh and not processed.

Since this diet is not a fast, getting regular exercise isn't a problem. This diet recommends about half-an-hour, six days a week. Full-body strength, interval training, cardio, and yoga are all recommended.

The diet is especially convenient for vegetarians and vegans, those who live gluten-free. Some of these organic and gluten-free ingredients will be more expensive than other foods, dieters should be warned. And as this is a hormone diet, hormone tests may be advisable to track progress and check for unexpected results. Those tests may not be covered by the dieter's insurance and could turn out to be rather costly.

This diet, like others, favors:

Cruciferous vegetables, which help livers metabolize the hormone estrogen and prevent estrogen-dominant cancers (Brussels sprouts, cauliflower, cabbage, kale, and bok choy)

Salmon and albacore tuna, which have the cholesterol needed to make male sex hormones such as testosterone and healthy omega-3 fatty acids, which help hormonal communication (Albacore tuna, flaxseed, walnuts, olive oil, chia seeds, avocados). Salmon also stabilizes the body's hunger hormones, controlling appetite

Avocados are rich in beta-sitosterol, to balance cortisol levels and positively affect cholesterol levels. Plant sterols influence progesterone and estrogen, hormones responsible for ovulation and menstrual cycle regulation.

Organic vegetables and fruits avoid the hormone-killing pesticides and chemicals like glyphosate, known endocrine-disrupters which reduce fertility, among other detrimental side-effects.

High-fiber carbohydrates (vegetables, fruits, whole grains) are known to clear out excess hormones, as well as facilitate chemical bonding and subsequent removal of active but unbound estrogens. Sweet potatoes, carrots, squashes, and other root vegetables are popular choice.

As we've discussed, probiotics are the so-called good bacteria in the gut. Prebiotics, on the other hand, are fibrous foods which those bacteria eat and thrive upon. To give you an idea of how important they are, the gut is the human body's largest endocrine organ. It creates and secretes over 20 hormones, each of which play a role in metabolism, appetite, and satiety (fullness). Prebiotic foods such as raw oats and garlic, dandelion, asparagus, apples, almonds, chicory, bananas, and Jerusalem artichokes. Kimchi and yogurt are rich in prebiotics as well.

On the other hand, there are foods which may only complicate a dangerous hormonal imbalance. They include fried foods, processed foods, sugar and sugar substitutes. These may ultimately impact the balance of the hormones ghrelin and leptin. Alcohol is a hormonal disrupter on a number of levels, from estrogen metabolism to blood sugar management.

So now we have a better idea of foods and how to use them, as that is truly what a diet is all about. But no diet protocol can cover every need your body will have. Not even the most clever dieter can get by just on the ketogenic diet or any other. Because as a diet progresses toward its target, especially in the early part of the diet, supplements may be crucial to success, even to survival. They're important during fasts, during diets and for overall wellness management. So lets take a look at the supplements you may be in desperate need of, some you may know well and some which will be entirely new to you.

Vegetarian and Vegan Diets

When well-planned, a vegetarian diet can be a very healthy way to meet daily nutritional needs. They continue to be popular for their various health benefits, including a reduction of risk of some cancers, diabetes, and heart disease.

They also parallel a lot of the other practices in this book, including fasting. And there are different kinds of vegetarian diets too, catering to different needs and different tastes. Lacto-vegetarian diets cut out fish, meats, eggs, poultry, but not dairy products such as cheese, milk, butter, and yogurt.

The ovo-vegetarian diet excludes meat, seafood, poultry, and dairy products, but it allow eggs. The lacto-ovo diet excludes fish, meat, and poultry, but it allows eggs and dairy products. Pescatarian diets exclude poultry meat, eggs, and dairy, but it does allow fish.

Vegan diets exclude poultry, eggs, meat fish, and dairy products, and all foods which contain any of these products.

The flexitarian diet is a plant-based diet, but it includes occasional, small portions of meat, dairy, eggs, poultry and fish.

A good vegetarian diet gets the most out of a spectrum of plant-based, healthy foods. Include fruits and vegetables, nuts and legumes, whole grains. Sugar-sweetened fruit juices and refined grains should be avoided.

This vegetarian diet offers daily portions based on 2,000-calorie diet Food group. As with all our recipes, observe the consistent measurements: vegetables and fruits at 1.5 – 2 cups (2 – 3 in these cases, as there is no meat in the diet), dressings to two tablespoons, pieces or slices of fruit and vegetables sides to between 1 and 5, salads at two cups of leafy greens. But here is where this diet differs, at his has significant grain and dairy portions which diets like the ketogenic diet do not have. Six and a half ounces of whole grains are recommended, dairy at three cups a day, protein foods at 3-4 ounces a day. The vegetarian diet also requires oils, from nuts or olives, at about 25-30 grams a day.

This diet, and the related vegan diet, also require a bit more supplementation, as they reduce or eliminate the natural sources of:

- Calcium and vitamin D: for strong bones and teeth, found in dark green vegetables, soy
- Vitamin B-12: necessary to producing red blood cells and preventing anemia
- Protein: maintains healthy bones, organs, muscles, and skin
- Omega-3 fatty acids: important for hearth health
- Iron and zinc: crucial for red blood cells
- Iodine: a vital component of thyroid hormones

Monday
- Breakfast: Overnight baked eggs bruschetta (baked in a casserole dish)
- Lunch: Arborio rice and white bean soup (arborio rice)
- Snacks: Cheese and fruit kabobs with yogurt
- Dinner: Grilled vegetarian pizza

Tuesday
- Breakfast: Shakshuka (poached eggs with onion, cumin, and tomatoes)
- Lunch: Roasted sweet potato salad with a honey-maple vinaigrette dressing
- Snack: Portobello bruschetta drizzled with rosemary aioli (caramelized onions and broiled peppers)
- Dinner: Vegetarian enchiladas (eggplant, corn, summer squash)

Wednesday
- Breakfast: Protein parfaits (yogurt, nuts, and fruit and nuts)
- Lunch: Mediterranean bulgur bowl (bulgur wheat, veggies, cheeses)

- Snack: Deviled eggs (with horseradish)
- Dinner: Lentil tacos

Thursday

- Breakfast: German Apple Pancake
- Lunch: Roasted sweet potato with chickpea pitas
- Snack: Stuffed mini peppers (with cheese and chives)
- Dinner: Pepper ricotta primavera (garlic, herbs, and pepper, ricotta cheese)

Friday

- Breakfast: Oatmeal waffles
- Lunch: Mozzarella-stuffed mushrooms and garlic toast
- Snack: Roasted beetroot with garlic hummus
- Dinner: Veggie pad Thai

Saturday

- Breakfast: Mushrooms Florentine (portobello)
- Lunch: Quinoa-stuffed squash (quinoa, garbanzo beans, pumpkin seeds)
- Snack: Chewy Honey Granola Bars

- Snack: Chewy Honey Granola Bars
- Dinner: Black bean tortilla pie

Sunday

- Breakfast: Black Bean & White Cheddar Frittata (with salsa, chipotle pepper)
- Lunch: Spinach quesadilla
- Snack: Homemade guacamole
- Dinner: Grilled bean burgers (garlic, cumin, chili powder)

Now here's a seven-day menu for those on a vegan diet. Note: For this diet plan, snacks should be limited to moderate portions of whole fruit or vegetables. Recipes should follow comparable recipes, or they'll be easy to find in many variations online.

Monday

- Breakfast: Mixed fruit smoothie
- Lunch: Hummus wrap
- Dinner: Spaghetti with shishito pepper and charred tomatoes and shishito peppers

Tuesday
- Breakfast: Peanut butter banana oatmeal
- Lunch: Portobello soup
- Dinner: Pizza burrito

Wednesday
- Breakfast: Avocado toast
- Lunch: Low-fat mashed chickpea sandwich (with vegetables)
- Dinner: Black bean enchilada burgers

Thursday
- Breakfast: Cacao smoothie
- Lunch: Black bean burrito
- Dinner: Low-fat taco bowl

Friday
- Breakfast: Berry Cobbler Overnight Oats
- Lunch: Balsamic spinach wrap (balsamic, salt, maple syrup, smoked paprika) over avocado and spinach
- Dinner: Pizza with veggies, chickpea sausage crumbles and creamy drizzle

Saturday
- Breakfast: Avocado pizza toast
- Lunch: Mediterranean wrap
- Dinner: Enchilada burrito

Sunday
- Breakfast: Banana split overnight oats
- Lunch: Flatbread with white bean puree with asparagus
- Dinner: Leftover easy black bean enchilada burger

CHAPTER TWELVE:
Natural Supplements

Our look into autophagy, fasting, weight loss, the molecular details of fats and cholesterol, and diets optimal health must now bring us to the realm of vital nutrients, vitamins, and minerals, and where to find them for your diet.

Holistic, organic, or natural healthcare may sound like far-out concepts, but chances are you or someone you know is already relying on it. According to the World Health Organization (WHO), 65 to 80 % of the global populace uses naturopathic, holistic medicine as their primary type of healthcare. In the United States alone, 38% of adults and even 12% of children have received one type of alternative medicine or another.

Keep in mind here that volumes have been written about these essential vitamins, minerals, herbs, and proteins. Each has a number of purposes, benefits, and side effects. As always, we strongly recommend you work closely with your specialist or physician before introducing anything new to your diet regiment. If there are any significant risks, we will include them here. But we will have to focus on the benefits as they relate to the subject of this book; fat burning, fasting, autophagy, hormonal balances. So while a lot of these nutrients may have benefits of other sorts, we're going to limit our study to the most relevant applications of each; weight loss, fat burning, fasting, and cellular regeneration.

Proteins, Enzymes, Vitamins, Minerals, Nutrients

Amino Acids: Amino acids are known as *the building blocks of all proteins*. They are intermediates in metabolism and must be ingested every day.

Beta-carotine: Beta-carotene is one of a group of natural chemicals known as carotenes or carotenoids. Beta-carotine boosts immunity and combats high blood pressure, its most applicable functions to our purposes here. It also aids immune-enhancing activity, proper cell communication, reproductive health, and is powerful antioxidant.

Vitamin B Complex: Vitamin B is compromised eight compounds: thiamine, niacin, riboflavin, folate, biotin, vitamin B6, folate, vitamin B12, and pantothenic acid and biotin: The vitamin B complex.

Thiamine: Thiamine (Vitamin B1) aids in the metabolism of carbohydrates and amino acids.

Riboflavin: Riboflavin (Vitamin B2) converts proteins, fats, and carbohydrates into energy.

Niacin: Niacin (Vitamin B3) helps synthesize fat and cholesterol, aids in the metabolism of carbohydrates, proteins and fat.

Pantothenic Acid and Biotin: Pantothenic Acid and Biotin (Vitamin B5 and vitamin B7) work together to convert carbohydrates, proteins and fats into energy.

Vitamin B-12: The body requires vitamin B12 for using certain amino acids and fatty acids which are essential to make DNA in your cells.

Vitamin B-6: Vitamin B-6 helps metabolize certain enzymes and make proteins. Vitamin B-5 helps to preserve normal immune and gastrointestinal function. Patients who are recovering from heart attacks are not advised to take vitamin B complex.

Conjugated Linoleic Acid: Conjugated Linoleic Acid (CLA) helps burn body fat, combat cardiovascular disease, fight high blood pressure, lower triglycerides and high cholesterol, boost insulin resistance and reduce inflammation.

Coenzyme Q10 (CoQ10): CoQ10 is an enzyme naturally found in every mitochondrial cell. About 95% of the body's energy is produced by these cells, converting fats and sugars into energy. Most of the body's CoQ10 is found in the internal organs, where they're needed most. CoQ10 is used to treat high blood pressure, obesity, diabetes, high cholesterol, heart disease, and immunity disfunction.

CoQ10 is an energizer and an antioxidant and energizer, preventing free radicals and scavenging for those already free.

Curcumin: Curcumin is an anti-inflammatory agent which as ant-carcinogenic, antioxidant, anti-inflammatory, and antimicrobial properties are exceeded by it's applications against gastrointestinal disorders, cardiovascular disease, gastrointestinal disorders, and liver disease. Curcumin is also a free radical scavenger and reduces free radical production. Curcumin has shown promise for cholesterol, treating diabetes and supporting heart health.

Vitamin C: Vitamin C promotes wound-healing and is to develop and maintain connective tissues like muscle and fat. It has anti-cholesterol and anti-diabetic qualities as well as being a powerful antioxidant and a booster to overall metabolism and detoxification.

Vitamin D: Vitamin D is used treat conditions of the heart and blood vessels, including high cholesterol and high blood pressure. It's beneficial for weight loss too, and is also used for a host of other conditions and diseases far too long to go into here.

Vitamin E: Vitamin E is popular for preventing and treating heart and blood vessel diseases including hardening of the arteries, heart attack, high blook pressure, diabetes, and other maladies. Vitamin E is sometimes used for improving physical endurance, increasing energy, reducing muscle damage after exercise. It is also an antioxidant.

Glutathione: Glutathione is recycled in the body, except when the toxic load becomes too great. Glutathione collects and cools off the free radicals and recycles other antioxidants.

All toxins cling onto glutathione, which carries them to the stool and the bile and out of the body. Higher glutathione levels reduce recover time, decrease muscle damage, and increase strength and endurance to shift metabolism away from fat production and toward muscle development.

Magnesium: Magnesium is essential to good health, the fourth most-abundant mineral in the human body. Approximately 50% of total body magnesium is found in bone. The other half is found predominantly inside cells of body tissues and organs. It maintains normal muscle function, heartbeat, regulate sugar levels and normal blood pressure. It may be connected to energy and protein metabolism.

Melatonin: Melatonin is a sleep aid, ideal for helping distracted fasters sleep through some hungry nights. It may also help with weight loss on its own. It's also used to treat high blood pressure and diabetes. Melatonin is possibly unsafe for use during pregnancy. Children should not use Melatonin.

Quercetin: Quercetin is a powerful antioxidant which may protect against heart disease, high blood pressure, respiratory infections.

Resveratrol: Resveratrol is an anti-inflammatory, antioxidant, anti-inflammatory substance found in red wine and dark chocolate, green teas, and some nuts. Resveratrol lowers cholesterol and protects against LDL oxidation. Resveratrol may also reduce inflammation, reverse obesity and diabetes and obesity. Resveratrol turns on a cell's natural survival pathways, Which prevents damage to individual cells. It may also aid in nutrient intake, weight loss, and remove accumulated toxins.

Zinc: Zinc, a metal, is known as an essential trace element, and is useful in treating type 2 diabetes.

Herbs

Alfalfa: Alfalfa is an excellent natural diuretic and laxative. It detoxifies the urinary tract and fights urinary tract infections. It's a very good neutralizer of intestinal acids and eases digestive problems including gastritis and indigestion. Alfalfa contains high levels of enzymes ideal for digestion. It may lower bad forms of cholesterol and stabilize blood sugar levels. Alfalfa Leaf is a powerful natural source of many essential vitamins including the entire complex of B-vitamins, A, E, D, E and K which is important for blood clotting.

Artichoke Leaf: Artichoke leaf treats chronic gastrointestinal and some gallbladder and liver conditions entailing high blood fat values. It's an antioxidant and choleretic.

Cascara Sagrada: Cascara Sagrada may improve the colon walls' musle tone in addition to its powers as laxative.

Corn Silk: Corn silk is used to treat diabetes, congestive heart failure, and high blood pressure.

Ginger: Ginger relieves gas pains, indigestion, stomach cramping, and diarrhea, It stimulates blood circulation, removing toxins and cleansing the kidney and bowels.

Pollen Extracts: Pollen extracts are known for their smooth muscle relaxation and anti-Inflammatory action.

Reishi: Red Reishi may enhance your immune system and improve your blood circulation. It's also used to high blood pressure, anxiety, high blood pressure, among other things.

And there's a virtual cookbook for necessary proteins, vitamins, nutrients, what they do and how to get them. Keep this chapter bookmarked for easy reference, as you may want to go back to it time and again. And when you're ready, you can move on to the other big step on your journey toward wellness. You've been through fasting, stimulating autophagy, defined our goals as to fat and cholesterol, chosen a diet, chosen the right supplements. Now it's time tor the next big step on your journey to total wellness.

Exercise.

SECTION 5: EXERCISE

CHAPTER THIRTEEN: Exercising During Fasts

We've looked at various sorts of fasting, the benefits and the risks. Some of our analyses have touched upon exercise, when it was well-advised and when it was not. We never recommend lethargy, but over-exertion when the body's resources are depleted can have dangerous and even deadly effects (on the heart, for example, as we've seen). There are risks, and there are benefits, and there are specific regiments which are better for some types of fasting than others. So let's take a closer look at this crucial part of a cleansing regiment and of a healthy lifestyle.

Exercising for Intermittent Fasting

Exercising is especially important when intermittent fasting. Because the dieter is still taking considerable amounts of calories (sometimes only half of their usual intake). That means their exercising regiment shouldn't be reduced by any more than half as well. In fact, exercise at this time will invigorate autophagy and reset the body for a more vigorous, energetic lifestyle. It also redirects the body's energies toward muscle growth, and muscle loss is a risk of fasting of any kind.

It's more than just the advantages of exercising during fasting, but the detriment to the body if one does not exercise during intermittent fasting.

Lethargy during fasting not only resets your body to a lethargic pace, but body reads this as a signal that the body is weak, too weak to manage a healthy fast (even if it is).

It tells your body you're too weak to handle a fast. In our paleolithic past, fasts were followed by a hunt, so this is what the body expects. Change your body's expectations and soon it will expect and deliver nothing but lethargy. Just as your body can reprogram itself during ketosis, it can reprogram its body during fasting. Lethargy tells the body not to develop body mass. That will have effects on hormonal production and begin a cycle of slowed metabolism, weight gain, and greater lethargy.

This can convince the dieter (just as the dieter has convinced their body) that fasting is unhealthy and to be abandoned. This, of course, only furthers more destructive habits of overeating, lethargy, imbalanced blood sugar levels, all the things which inspired the decision to fast in the first place. The dieter has also taken one of their most potent weapons for longevity off the table, psychologically speaking at least.

Weight lifting is, by and large, a good exercise for fasting, as it focuses on muscle development. They're great for intermittent fasting, as there are always enough biological resources to divert attention toward muscle growth.

During intermittent fasting, general daily exercise is almost certainly adequate, perhaps even optimal. The body is already going through some extreme changes with the fasting, it doesn't need extreme physical exertion as well. Anything up to twenty-four hours in considered intermittent, and whatever the preferred mode of exercise is, it should suffice. Walking is always a good moderate form of exercise, though it's not very intense. Jogging is a bit higher impact, though anybody should check with their doctor before starting a jogging regiment. It can be hard on the joints and the heart. And since fasting can deplete essential minerals like calcium, care should be taken before running for extended periods.

Moderate calisthenics such as sit-ups, push-ups and pull-ups are also idea for exercise during intermittent fasting.

But some intermittent fasting requires abstinence (from caloric intake) for more than 24 hours, so they require a bit more of a deliberate application for maximum effectiveness and minimal risk. The longer the fast, the more care needs to be taken.

1. Walking: For longer periods of fasting, walking is all the more important as a form of exercise. It works muscle groups for growth, it burns calories, it instigates autophagy, increases

metabolism. The movement is good for digestion. It's good for the circulatory and respiratory systems, and helps clear toxins out of the body through perspiration and, later, urination and bowel movements.

Walking is also an excellent distraction. It gives a dieter time to think about other things besides fasting (and how hungry they are). Walking is famous for its opportunities to reflect, to think about other important things in life; social relationships, career challenges, plans for the future. Walking has a famously meditative quality, a calming effect that we'll look at in greater detail shortly.

Morning walks in particular are recommended during fasting. In fact, the fasted morning walk is an old bodybuilder trick for cutting body fat. The idea is to consume no calories before the walk and let the body use only reserves. After fasting through the night, the body will be ready to start using its resources. A fasted jog or even a cycle session forces body fat our of reserve and into circulation, to be expelled. Insulin is also generally low in the morning, aiding if fat burning.

2. Weights: As we've said briefly, lifting weights is a great way to preserve muscle during longer fasts. Strategies for weight lifting differ depending on whether the dieter is fasting intermittently or long-term.

And, as we've said, the longer the fast, the more care has to be taken with exercise. So if you're fasting for 16 hours at a time, just go on lifting weights as you might normally do. Think about upping your reps, if you feel comfortable doing it.

But here are some tips if you're doing fasting for longer periods and you're concerned about muscle loss:

- Lift at higher intensities to lower the amount of reps in a single cycle
- Don't lift to failure (lifting until the final rep can't be completed)
- Don't max-out your repetitions during a longer-term fast

- Don't max-out on effort either. On a one-to-ten scale, keep it somewhere between six and eight
- Favor full-body exercises over isolated reps.

The whole body is undergoing autophagy, the cells and muscles of every part of the body are affected. So it only makes sense to spread that energy equally over every part of the body. And remember that fasting resets the body, and you don't want to instruct your body to focus on one part at the expense of the others. Your weightlifting regiment should match that.

Cardio: While fasting, so-called *easy cardio* is ideal, especially for extended fasts. And the longer the fasting goes, the easier the dieter should go with the exercise. Cardio is shorthand for endurance training, which is idea for fasting (which requires its own kind of endurance). During a long-term fast, keep your cardio intensity in the so-called *aerobic zone*, the heart rate at which the body is burning calories primarily from body fat. It's a moderate-to-high heart rate, but one which is sustainable and not overly intense. There's a handy equation to find your ideal aerobic heart rate: Your age subtracted from 180. If you're 50 years old, your ideal aerobic rate of beats per minute is 130. If you're 20 years old, your ideal beats per minute (BPM) is 160. Don't exceed these BPMs if you're fasting.

You won't feel overly taxed, which is good. That means your body is using fat as fuel, the easy way, instead of increased sugar cravings or using glycogen stores.

When fasts get longer, stay away from intense endurance training. Sprinting and jogging are likewise not recommended.

But it's not just what you eat, but when you eat it. All of the diets we recommended suggest regular eating times. And when you're exercising, that should be timed in correlation to eating windows.

Even during short-term fasting, you'll want to time your workouts a bit more deliberately. One study demonstrated that males on eating-window regiments who lifted to failure eight to twelve reps over four sets consumed 650 less calories than those who were not observing fasting eating windows. They retained and even improved muscle mass. However, the non-fasting group showed greater size gains.

A study in women found resistance training let to muscle gains even on a time-restricted eating schedule, as long as intake of protein and calories were maintained.

Most specialists suggest not breaking a fast immediately after a workout to augment the release of growth hormone, which burns fat and maintains tissues.

Exercise During Long-term Fasting

The longer you fast, the more careful you have to working out, right? So let's take a closer look at the potentially dangerous practice.

First, let's go back to the other caveat about fasting and working out. The longer you've been fasting, the less you want to exert yourself. It's also worth pointing out here (once again) that if muscle-building is your goal, fasting may not be your best approach. If you hope to slim down and then bulk up, fasting will help slim you down and working out will help you bulk up, those are two consecutive goals, each with a proper strategy, not one goal with an improper strategy.

If your goal is to maintain muscle mass during a fast (a good idea) then your reps and cycles and weight intensity should only be in accordance with the duration and intensity of the fast. If you're fasting a bit longer, lift a bit less. But do lift, as it prevents lethargy and atrophy. Consider a regiment of one to two days a week of full-body workouts while intermittent fasting.

Time workouts for the middle of an eating window so you can go home and have a good meal and replenish your nutrients.

Fasted cardio, which we touched on briefly before, is a favorite of athletes who are fasting. Their morning hours for fasted cardio are usually between seven and ten in the morning.

You may never have wondered what actually happens to fat when you exercise. As we've seen, stored glycogen is the first choice for the body's energy. After about a half-hour to an hour, the body begins burning fat.

Experts recommend at least 30 minutes of cardio two to three times a week. For weight loss and proper management, physical activity of up to an hour a day is often recommended, given normal dietary and medicinal intake.

(Remember to act responsibly with these or any exercises and consult your doctor.)

An Important Note

This is crucial for using this book from this point forward. We're about to start introducing exercises into this book, to use the knowledge you're accumulating and put it to real, physical use. Here, as they say, is when we start putting boots on the ground (or hands on the matt, as it were). And up until now, the likelihood is that you've been reading this book as a solitary endeavor (the way most books are written). But while you can read the upcoming exercise or yoga instructions and memorize them, that will be in conflict to the very goals of those applications. And nobody I've ever known could read and meditate at the same time. The two things are practically antithetical. And you certainly can't read to yourself during hypnosis.

So we have two recommendations for implementing the applications which are to follow. The idea is that you'll need somebody reading these yoga courses while you perform them, you'll need a voice to guide you while you meditate and during hypnosis.

One choice is to record your voice. It's as easy as downloading a smartphone voice recording app. Read the directions for the exercises and practices into the app and play them back for yourself. This frees you up to clear your mind and perform the often-complex maneuvers which these practices sometimes require. The benefits of this approach are: Convenience, since nobody else needs to be inconvenienced by your workouts; privacy, which fasters, dieters, and self-care practitioners crave and deserve; and self-control, since you can record the directions at the pace which suits you.

The drawbacks to this approach are that you lack the input of somebody who can see what you're doing wrong. That objective viewpoint is something you will be harder pressed to do for yourself, even with an adequate mirror.

These things do often require a certain amount of expertise to avoid injury and maximize the benefits. That's why so many people see yogis, exercise trainers, meditation coaches. Each of these schools have their own subtleties and challenges and many of us just don't know enough to work our way through it, DIY.

It's also a bit isolating, which it is sometimes meant to be. Other times, group support is helpful and even necessary.

Another approach is to include a second person in your workouts and meditations (and especially hypnosis). They don't have to be experts, as we'll provide the expertise. They just have to be willing and able. This approach has a lot of benefits and a few drawbacks too.

A second person provides support, encouragement, and perhaps expertise. But a second person can also improvise and contribute a perspective which no prerecorded voice can do. It's flexible, and flexibility is key to the systems we're manipulating and the way in which we manipulate them.

There is also the presence of a second person, which can't be underestimated. Feelings of isolation may lead to a sense of weakness, helplessness, and that may discourage further application.

It is also reciprocal in its own way. After your partner guides you on an exercise or a yoga session, you can turn around and guide them. That will only increase your understanding, even mastery of these techniques. This will give you the objective perspective you necessarily lack when engaged in your own exercises and applications. Having a partner means you can be a partner.

Drawback include convenience. A lot of people like you and me just don't have a second person on hand at all times of the day or night. A lot of these exercises require a certain amount of juggling to work into your schedule. Working them into two different schedules can be more than twice as difficult.

Also, you shouldn't be relying on anyone else for your progress. This is about you and you alone, at least at first. After you've made some progress you can help others, but the onus is on you to take those first steps, and you just may have to take them alone. If you do, you can still make the most of it.

In point of fact, your pursuit of these things may naturally take you from an isolated practice to one filled with support. Individual exercises will likely draw you to classes, to other like-minded people whom you can work with to achieve your mutual ends.

Either way, it would take a stone-cold genius to read and memorize these instructions and then instruct themselves while practicing to optimal effect. If that's you, congratulations! If not, start to think now about how you're going to help yourself through the more complex exercises and applications you're about to face.

But don't be discouraged by this. Don't be tempted to believe that you've gone as far as you can go and just give up. See it as an opportunity to reach out to others, to increase your social circle, to help others and to learn to accept help when its offered. These are milestones toward greater wellness on their own, even being willing to admit that help is needed is a significant step forward for you and any one you know.

For now, there's still a bit more reading to do. Finish the book, familiarize yourself with what will be expected of you. Educate yourself. You may want to get a support friend or an exercise partner after you've finished reading. You may want that person to read this book to, so you're on the same page (if you'll pardon that expression). Of, if you can't wait, then download a voice recording app (to your laptop or desktop or tablet if you don't have a smartphone), roll up your sleeves, and prepare to get down to it.

Exercise Apps

Before you follow our exercise instructions, be aware that we're far from the only source of such things. In fact, we suggest use of apps and other books, videos, anything that will help you along on your journey to full-body wellness. Here are the best ones we could find online, and what they have to offer. Keep in mind that, as with all our lists of apps, detox kits, or any other product, we have no connection to any of them. We are not endorsing any specific brand or product, simply giving you the best information we can find to help you make the best decisions you can.

Keep in mind that, unlike previous apps, these apps are not all free. Some of them are quite pricey, actually.

Apple Fitness Plus is truly the head of the pack when it comes to monitoring your exercising via computer electronics. The subscription fitness service works for the watch and other devices such as the iPhone. The subscription is $9.99 per month.

PEAR Personal Fitness Coach is free and available for Android or iOS and it's free, but the subscription is $5.99 per month. Its specialties include:

- Hands-free, eyes-free audio coaching
- Guided workouts at a variety of levels.
- Wide variety of workout packages
- Performance tracking
- Sharing with other apps

Fitbit Coach is available for Android and iOS for a subscription of $39.99 per year or $7.99 per month. It allows the user to:

Log daily activities

Recommend exercise activities

Enjoy dynamic workouts which intuitively increase in difficulty according to input

Workout Trainer, free for Android and iOS: Free, plus different subscription rates starting at $6.99 per month). It offers:

- Training routines and exercises for newbies and veterans.
- A simple questionnaire
- Recommended workout plans and exercises personalized to the user's fitness goals.
- Reminders and notifications
- Streak tracking
- Stat tracking
- One-on-one trainers hired for various fitness specialties.

Peloton is available for Android and iOS for $12.99/£12.99 monthly. This app helps you conveniently (and safely) take advantage of what Peloton offers without the expensive (and allegedly dangerous) treadmill. The app is:

- Free to download
- Offers a 30-dayfree trial

- Guided workouts in just about everything from cardio to yoga to stretching.
- Group workouts
- Tag joining

Fit Radio, for Andriod and IOs, has a number of unique features:

- It generates new playlists for every workout, designed to inspire.
- It serves different workouts from ellipticals to bike rides to low-density to high-density interval training
- Seven-day free trial ($9.99 after that)

Shred is available for Android and iOS for $12.99 monthly. As the name suggests, it's a favorite of fans of intense workouts. This is a good supplemental app to a traditional gym workout. Some benefits of the app are:

- Workout types options (bodyweight, gym, cardio)
- Shred community
- Interactive visuals
- Activity logging

- 7-day free trial

Seven, free for Android and iOS, offers:

- Seven-minute-a-day training
- Connection to friends to track progress
- 3D guides
- Subscription Seven Club ($9.99 monthly or $79.99 annually)

JEFIT is free to download for Android and iOS and specializes in bodybuilding and strength training. Special features include:

- Thousands of routines
- Routines sorted by target body part
- Detailed instructions
- Workout planner
- Progress tracker
- Exercise log

Belly Fat Exercises

1. Burpees: This is a great exercise for the core, and also for the chest, lats, shoulders, quads,

triceps. In involves explosive plyometric movement and will get your heart pumping!

Note: When you do these exercises, the beginning stance is generally with your feel shoulder-distance apart. In other words, each foot is precisely under its corresponding shoulder.

So, with the burpee, you'll stand (feet being shoulder-distance apart) and push your hips back. Lower your body in a slow, low squat. Put your hands flat on the floor just outside of where your feet are. Then quickly push your feet back and straighten out, letting your chest touch (but not rest) on the floor. Push your hands flat and lift your body into a plank. Now reverse it and pull your feet back to where your hands are and stand up, all just as fast as you did the first half. The explosive nature of the cycle is crucial to its effectiveness. The move includes elements of the push-up and the power-squat.

Some people accentuate this exercise by holding a medicine ball. It's held in the hands at first before being lowered and left on the floor through the planking portion of the exercise, then picked up and raised at the end of the rotation.

2. Mountain Climbers: Like burpees, this moving plank exercise works a variety of muscle groups but focuses on the core.

Get into the same high-plank position you used for Berpees, wrists directly under the shoulders. Keeping the core tight, draw the belly button inward toward the spine. Drive the right knee inward toward the chest, then return the foot back to straighten the leg, bringing it back to the plank position. Then drive the left knee inward toward the chest, then return the leg to plank. Alternate right and left sides as many rounds as you wish.

3. Overhead medicine ball slams are great for the core, for endurance, for the heart rate. The heaviest ball you can manage, the better.

Stand with your feet hip-width apart (instead of shoulder width) and hold the medicine ball tightly with both hands. Stretch both arms up over your head, stretching your body. Slam the ball down and forward and down, bending your knees slightly as you hinge forward. Squat a bit to pick up the ball and stand again. Raising the ball again starts the cycle again.

4. Russian twists are great for the core and also improve definition and strength.

Start by sitting on the ground in a sit-up position, a medicine ball in both hands held at the chest. Raise your feet up off the floor, lean back to a 45-degree angle. Twist your torso right and left while holding the medicine ball in both hands, keeping your feet above the floor.

5. Running on an incline is a great way to burn fat. Running itself is good cardio, but an incline may increase that burn by as much as 50%. You might try start off with a walk or jog for five or ten minutes, then start jogging or even running. There's a lot of benefit to slowing to a walk for five to then, then jogging from five to ten, then alternating again. As you get stronger, consider extending the running portions of this rotation to twenty or thirty minutes or more, keeping the walking stretches to ten or even decreasing them to no more than five.

6. Rowing machines are a great way to work up the heart rate, burn calories and melt fat while you build muscles in the back, shoulders, arms, legs and core.

Here's an effective 4-minute cycle: Start with 20 seconds' rowing and ten seconds' rest. Remain in the rowing position when at rest, and note the miles or meters traveled. Repeat the cycle eight times, each time trying to improve your distance. After the eight rest, go for a quick 500 meters and see how long that takes. Try to beat this number the next time.

7. HIIT is based on the idea that short bursts of intense cardio are best for burning fat, as opposed to sustained periods of lower-intensity cardio.

After a 10-minute warm-up, do 30 seconds of as many repetitions as you can manage of any one thing: Push-ups, squats, single-arm rows, or kettlebell swings. Rest for 30 seconds and choose a different exercise for another 30-second round. Do this for ten rounds, ten different exercises. Make sure you choose the exercises to work different muscle groups.

8. Strength Training is a good way to lose weight too. While most weight lifting isn't designed to burn fat exclusively (that may be the goal but the effect is merely secondary). While moderately heavy weights are usually used for cardio or weight management, and very heavy lifting is designed for putting on muscle mass, there is an area in between which is perfect for burning fat.

If you're not lifting any weights, get some and start lifting; just a few hand weights at home will do the trick. If you're already lifting, increase the weight and duration of your workouts. This creates the afterburn effect, wherein fat is being burned even after the workout is over.

9. Walking has appeared before on our list of exercises for a variety of things, and that should come as no surprise. Walking is good for the body and the mind. It's good for metabolism, for autophagy, for virtually every system in the body.

Experts recommend between 45 and 60 minutes of brisk walking daily to improve metabolism. It also may prevent overtraining. Overtraining may lead to an excessive production of cortisol, the stress hormone which contributes to belly fat. Experts suggest that one hour's worth of rapid walking per day may generate one lost pound of fat per week.

From diet to exercise, our journey can only take us to one logical place, and that's Yoga. Yoga and fasting interconnect in a number of intriguing and educational ways. The mind and body have been getting closer and closer, from autophagy to fasting and then the rest, it's all been a long and complex intermingling of mind and body, with the mind continuously guiding the body toward more effective autophagy and greater overall wellness.

And, looking ahead, our next step will take us naturally to the one after that. At this point, it's important to note how one thing builds upon the one before it, and prepares one for what is next to come. This is why the stages aren't to be skipped, at least not in the first reading. Everything is mindful and deliberate to deliver you to the future you envision for yourself, which we'll get to in greater detail later.

For now, it's onward and upward (literally) into the world of yoga as it relates to fasting and the dietary practices you've been implementing. So unroll your matt, stretch out, and open your mind and your heart … and your hips. It's yoga time.

SECTION 6: YOGA FOR FASTING

CHAPTER FOURTEEN:
Yoga for Fasting

Fasting Meets Yoga

Yoga and fasting actually have a lot in common. Each entail a great deal of discipline and physical stamina. Both are good for physical fitness and psychological wellness. Yoga requires the kind of meditative mindset which is critical to a successful fast, as we have seen.

And both are centered around the idea of detachment, or rising above the daily scurry of life to achieve a higher physical and mental state.

Both yoga and fasting ask us to resist temptation, to eschew instant gratification. If yoga is your principle focus, your main challenge may be to overcome lethargy and stay on the map. If fasting is your course, your challenges may be focused around your efforts to overcome hunger. Yoga is great for either, and there are certain yoga regiments for a fasting-friendly approach.

As we know, fasting allows our digestive functions to rest and to reinvigorate. Most of us run our systems around the clock and never think twice about it, much less give it a deliberate rest. But this book is all about being deliberate, being mindful.

There's another connection between fasting and yoga which makes them go perfectly together. Fasting rids the body of a lot of extra mass, either water weight or accumulated fecal matter, or fat reserves around the belly. Fasting for any duration rids the body of these obstructive weights. True, it takes more than fasting or yoga to keep the weight off, the loss of the weight makes the body more flexible, more capable of the elasticity yoga requires. And yoga, in return, stretches the muscles and keeps them growing, essential during a fast.

Fasting also has meditative qualities, as we've discussed. It calls upon users to recalibrate their relationships with food, and with our needs and desires to eat. It gives a faster more time to walk and to think about other things, if for no other reason than to distract the mind from the belly.

A lot of fasting is religious, some of it political. It's main purpose in these cases is to focus the mind by focusing the body. But the benefits of fasting are much broader, paving the way toward deeper states of awareness. All the world's major religions feature some form of fasting. Jews fast during Yom Kippur, Christians deny themselves certain things during the Lenten period before Easter Sunday, Muslims have Ramadan. In the lineage of Tantra Yoga, one of the niyamas has a direct relation to food consumption. Inspya Yoga's teacher training requires a ten-day detox.

Politically, Bobby Sands drew worldwide attention to the plight of the Irish Republican Army in the early 1980s. In 2021, Russian anti-Putin protestor Alexi Navalny staged a hunger strike after being arrested in Moscow.

But it's the spiritual realization of fasting which is particularly potent when it comes to yoga. Even when not in a spiritual or religious context, fasting brings mental clarity. We know this because of the autophagy which happens in the brain, improving performance (as it does for every organ). And that clearing of the mind is the hand and yoga is the key to unlock that spiritual realization.

As it is with fasting and diet and exercise, all things work together for the improvement of the whole in a well-balanced system.

So yoga can give the faster strength even as the faster brings improved flexibility. Focus and strength improve in both areas of life.

Both yoga and fasting give a person a feeling of accomplishment as well, verifiable and even immediate rewards for the efforts. The body feels better during and after yoga, as it does during and after a period of fasting (either short- or long-term).

Yoga is also right in line with intermittent fasting. In yoga, the suggested break between meals is a full eight hours. (This is to allow the excretory system to function properly.) That's breakfast, dinner, and no lunch. This is already one of the favored types of intermittent fasts we read about earlier. Just another way fasting and yoga seem to go hand-in-hand. In fast, fasting is a very common practice among yogis.

Yoga embraces various long-term fasting techniques, including water and juice fasts, as well as dry fasts for up to several days. A healthy person can manage a wet fast for up to five days. As long as or more than seven days is not recommended for anyone.

Here are a few tips to keep your yoga regiment going smoothly while you're fasting.

While motion is key to yoga, and some physical activity is important to fasting, there will be times when you may feel too weak or unmotivated for a lot of energetic movement which is sometimes required of yoga. In that case, and these may strike during a fast, there is always *seva* (selfless service or karma yoga), *pranayama* (breathing exercises), meditation and concentration. You might even spend some time simply reading and learning about yoga, which is definitely a part of the practice (and perfect if you just don't have the energy). If you find you consistently lack the energy for even a mild yoga session, you may be following a regiment lacking in proteins, healthy carbs, or healthy fats.

Make sure the timing is right for you. You may be choosing the wrong time of day or the wrong day of the week. Remember that timing and regularity are important in working out while fasting, and the same applies here. If you're consistently lacking in energy in the evenings, you may want to get up early and do your yoga sessions before the work day begins. If you're skipping lunch during your eight-hour fasting window between meals (a yogi practice as we've seen) you may spend your lunch hour doing yoga. If your work days are simply too busy with other things, you may consider doubling up on your yoga sessions on the weekends. If you're too tired from your work week and your diet is adequate, you may be working too hard. Meditation may be a good alternative to yoga, one we'll look at shortly.

If you're committing to a yoga regiment, start slow. If you're new to it, find some guidance if you can. There are lots of classes for people at different levels and it should be easy to find the right class for your level, location, and schedule. But don't get locked into a slower regiment. The whole idea of fasting, dieting, yoga, meditating, any of the practices we discuss, is to keep going with them, to let your practices evolve as you evolve. The more you need, the more you should take. The less you can handle, the more you should leave on the table.

Beginners may start with a couple of rounds of sun salutation and five or so other poses of choice, and investigating more static and gentler practices like Yin Yoga (where in each pose is held for between three and ten minutes). Yin Yoga is ideal for releasing connective bands and tissues around the muscles. This provides a better opportunity for the body to relax, promoting circulation and clearly blockages.

These practices help reduce *tamas* (darkness, chaos) and *rajas* (passion, confusion) and promote *sattva* (purity). So fasting may include keeping one's surroundings and one's body clean, abstaining from lying or gossip, controlling negative emotions such as anger and a cranky mood.

Some *Pranayama* (breathing exercises) which can be easily perform while fasting include Diaphragmatic Breathing (yogic breathing), which calms the mind and brings focus in times of distraction. Another is *Bhramari Pranayama* (bee breath) for a deepen of concentration and preparation for meditation.

Here are other good poses for yogic fasting:

- *Bhujangasana* (Cobra pose)
- *Setu Bandhasana* (Bridge pose)
- *Balasana* (Child's pose)
- *Ardha matsyendrasana* (Seated spinal twist)
- *Paschimottanasana* (Seated forward fold)
- *Shavasana* (Corpse pose for relaxation)

Admittedly, this is hardly an encyclopedia of yoga terms and positions. Entire books have been written on that subject, and you're well-advised to get one, preferably an illustrated book (there are lots of them). But we hope you've achieved a working knowledge of what yoga is, why you might be doing it, and how to get the most out of it while fasting. We've also tried to show how yoga will help you get the most out of fasting.

Before we put all that to use on your body and mind, let's take a quick look at popular yoga apps.

Yoga Apps

Yoga Studio is a top-ranked yoga app which has a number of impressive benefits, including:
- High-quality content
- Ease of use
- Excellent value
- Numerous custom classes
- Focus on balance, flexibility, strength, and relaxation
- Ideal for back pain
- Custom flow creation
- Schedule and track classes
- Library of over 280 poses
- Choose or create music tracks

- Subscriptions by the week

Down Dog is also popular, mostly for these features:
- Useful as you progress
- Routines and lessons for all levels
- Different practice durations (from ten minutes to 110)
- Generates new sequences

Daily Yoga specializes in community motivation and support. It's most popular features include:
- Weekly activities for motivation
- 200 guided yoga classes, 500 asanas, 50 work out plans (with subscription)
- Multi-week programs
- Constant additions of new videos and programs

Glo is a popular app for yogis and those who are too busy for regular studio classes. It offers:
- Five-, Ten-, or 20-minute classes
- User friendly app

- Challenging and beginner friendly classes

Simply Yoga is great for kids (and adults) who are at the beginner level. It offers:

- Sequences of 20, 40, or even 60 minutes
- Easy-to follow instructions
- 21-day or 30-day challenges

That should be enough info to get you started on finding the best yoga app. Now let's put this knowledge into some serious practice with a specially designed program for yoga during fasting.

CHAPTER FIFTEEN: A Program for Yoga During Fasting

We're already seen the benefits of periodic fasting. And practicing yoga only amplifies the power of the resets of autophagy which comes about during fasting. So here is a program to cleanse the mind and the body in more powerful ways.

As always, the usual caveat apply: Consult a doctor, follow prescribed guidelines, do not strain yourself to the point of injury.

This program is flexible. If you're planning a one day fast, just practice the first day's exercises. Feel your way through the week and stop if you feel you need to. Both yoga and fasting require gradual assimilation, and that's even more important when you're doing both at once. Re-evaluate after your third day, if you get that far, and see if you shouldn't take a break in your fast and repeat those three days the following week, to take it further then if you feel up to it. Good change is gradual change.

This program is a three-, four-, or five-day program wherein you remove a food from your diet and add a yoga practice in its place. The duration is flexible upon the user's requirements and abilities.

This program offers two yoga classes from which to choose, one more rigorous and one more gentle. The rigorous classes gradually decrease in intensity as energy reserves decrease. But one body may be more energetic one day and less so the next, so the options make the most of this natural tendency. And if you repeat the program, you can switch every class from the one you did the cycle before, giving you an almost-endless combination of classes in any given week. Remember to do one class per day only, don't try to do two or three options in a single day.

The program also includes a meditation option for each day, as meditation is an important part of what yoga and fasting are all about. And just as being active helps to properly reset the body after autophagy, meditation resets the mind on the right track in the same way. We will look at such meditative practices as they relate to fasting in the next chapter, but they belong here as part of the week-long program.

This program is ideal for those interested in the mental and physical benefits of fasting, beginning and advanced yoga practitioners, and anyone interested in complimenting their health regiment with yoga.

Note that the program entails one yoga position after the next, but we also understand that you might not know all the positions by name. So we'll lean toward describing the action and naming the positions when we can.

Day 1

Gentle Option: Toxic Twist

This detox class is first exercise for a reason; it's great for setting the body's reset button. It's hard work and really gets your juices flowing to kickstart a new detoxification regiment.

Twisting the body cleanses the liver and the kidneys. And there are plenty of twists in this class in different variations and with different variations. Drink plenty of water during and particularly after the toxic twist or its more rigorous option.

Start with a downward-facing dog position, which is feet and hands on the floor, legs straight, head down. Exhale. Lower your body flat on the floor, touching down before curling your spine to lift your head up, hands on the floor at the sides of your chest. This is the tall cobra position. Arch your back and raise your head, inhaling, then lower back down while you raise your up off the floor. Keep your knees and hands on the floor, arms straight, head down, breathing deeply. Then return to downward-facing dog pose again.

Raise the left leg up behind you as far as you can, keeping the leg straight and the toes extended. Then bring your left leg back and all the way in, touching your left knee to your chest, hands still on the ground. Left foot on the floor, lift up your body, raising your hands above your head. Lower your hands to your heart and look down.

Put your right hand on the floor and twist to reach up with your left hand as you exhale. Hold and stretch, then return your left hand to the floor as you exhale. Return your right hand to the floor and straighten your right leg back. Return to the downward-facing dog position.

Exhale and straight your body as you lower your belly and chest to the floor, exhaling. Curl your back up in tall cobra position, hands flat on the floor as you pull yourself up, spine arching, head back, inhaling. Hold that position.

As you exhale, keeping your hands and knees on the floor, push yourself back, facing down. Your weight is on your calves in this position, you knees wide apart. Turn your palms upward to twist your arms and shift your hips a little to one side, then the other.

Now we'll do the same to the right side.

Raise the right leg up behind you as far as you can, keeping the leg straight and the toes extended. Then bring your right leg back and all the way in, touching your right knee to your chest, hands still on the ground. right foot on the floor, lift up your body, raising your hands above your head. Lower your hands to your heart and look down.

Put your left hand on the floor and twist to reach up with your right hand as you exhale. Hold and stretch, then return your right hand to the floor as you exhale. Return your left hand to the floor and straighten your right leg back. Return to the downward-facing dog position.

Exhale and straight your body as you lower your belly and chest to the floor. Curl your back up in tall cobra position, hands flat on the floor as you pull yourself up, spine arching, head back, inhaling. Hold that position.

As you exhale, keeping your hands and knees on the floor, push yourself back, spine parallel to the floor, head facing down. Your weight is on your calves in this position, you knees wide apart. Turn your palms upward to twist your arms and shift your hips a little to one side, then the other.

Repeat as desired.

Rigorous Option: Soft Heart with A Twist; Chaturanga Free Practice

Trusting our legs and core to be strong, yoga allows the heart to be oft. The movement to ease the heart space is the backbend. Twists and side bends expand space in the ribcage and in the heart. This practice is wrist-friendly.

Start with arms up, knees slightly bent. Lower the body to rest on the knees. Bring the right knee forward and up, foot on the floor and raise the left arm up straight. Then lean to the right, stretching your left arm as you breathe deeply. Hold that position.

Then twist and lower your right arm to touch your right elbow to the outside of your left knee. Your left hand is pointing up toward the ceiling, palm flat. Now raise your right arm and place your right hand flat against your left, palm-to-palm. Allow your right hip to move toward your left knee.

Press your left elbow into your right knee. Turn your face rightward toward the ceiling and look up. Expand the capacity of your lungs, the capacity of your heart. Exhale. Straighten your spine and reach up, arms straight. Lower your hands, palms to the floor as the left knee rises. Inhale as you half-lift your body, right leg straight, toes and fingertips on the floor.

Bring your feet together, legs slightly bent at the knees. Exhale as you lean fully forward and drop your head, hands touching the floor by your feet. Reach up and stand, legs slightly bent as before. Legs still bent, lower your arms and then reach back behind you (the airplane position).

Bring your arms forward and then up in front of you until they're reaching straight up to the ceiling and, in the same motion, raise your right leg. Find your balance at the outside of your left foot. Allow your right hip to descend, twist to the right with your left arm in front and your right arm stretched out behind you. Reach down with your left hand and press it against the outside of your upraised right knee, your right arm still outstretched behind you. Pull your right knee in with your left hand. You may choose to let your left arm float, that will work the core even more.

Release and return to a standing position, facing forward. Return to the original position, arms upraised and knees slightly bent.

Now do the same for the other side.

Start with arms up, knees slightly bent. Lower the body to rest on the knees. Bring the left knee forward and up, foot on the floor and raise the right arm up straight. Then lean to the left, stretching your right arm as you breathe deeply. Hold that position.

Then twist and lower your left arm to touch your left elbow to the outside of your right knee. Your right hand is pointing up toward the ceiling, palm flat. Now raise your left arm and place your left hand flat against your right, palm-to-palm. Allow your left hip to move toward your right knee. Press your right elbow into your left knee. Turn your face leftward toward the ceiling and look up. Expand the capacity of your lungs, the capacity of your heart. Exhale. Straighten your spine and reach up, arms straight. Lower your hands, palms to the floor as the right knee rises. Inhale as you half-lift your body, left leg straight, toes and fingertips on the floor.

Bring your feet together, legs slightly bent at the knees. Exhale as you lean fully forward and drop your head, hands touching the floor by your feet. Reach up and stand, legs slightly bent as before. Legs still bent, lower your arms and then reach back behind you (the airplane position).

Bring your arms forward and then up in front of you until they're reaching straight up to the ceiling and, in the same motion, raise your left leg. Find your balance at the outside of your right foot. Allow your left hip to descend, twist to the left with your right arm in front and your left arm stretched out behind you. Reach down with your right hand and press it against the outside of your upraised left knee, your left arm still outstretched behind you. Pull your left knee in with your right hand. As with the other side, you may choose to let your right arm float, that will work the core even more.

Release and return to a standing position, facing forward. Return to the original position, arms upraised and knees slightly bent.

Repeat as desired.

Meditative Option: Meditate & Cultivate Calm

This 15-minute-long meditation is perfect for beginners and advanced meditators and anyone in between. The practice focuses on enjoying the meditative process without getting hung up on meditating correctly. Remaining connected to the breath will make you will feel calmer, lighter, and clearer.

Sit comfortably with your legs crossed, knees out and ankles in. A good tip to have your knees in line with your hips, or even lower. That's central to the lotus position, to keep the knees low. Use a pillow or yoga block for greater comfort if you like. Place your hands on your knees with palms up, take a deep breath, Feel your tailbone lower, as if it were connected to the earth. Then feel your heart rise up, through your head and up as if it were connected to the heavens.

Take a deep breath brough your nose and right into your heart center. Relax your shoulders and exhale.

Repeat as desired.

Day 2

Gentle Option: Reset Refuge; Bliss Out and Be Blessed

Experience the bliss of this smooth and soft and practice. This class combine hip openers and gentle flow, self-massage, twists, *mudra* and *pranayama* and enhance the body, soul, and mind.

Stand on your knees, facing forward. Pull the right knee back to a 45-degree angle behind you, pelvis lowered, right leg in front and bent at the knee, foot on the floor. Lean back and inhale while extending your arms to your sides, then bending the elbows to raise the hands upright at the sides of your head. Keep your elbows at a point behind your shoulders.

Set your left hand on the left knee and twist, bringing your right arm across to the left side of your body. Bend the right arm and press the right elbow against the outside of the left knee. Make a fist with your right hand and cover it with your left hand, left elbow up. With the right elbow against the left knee, twist to the left with greater force. Turn your torso up and toward the left. Take a deep breath right in to the belly and then slowly and gracefully release. Don't rush that.

Walk (or inch) your left foot toward the right, then lower yourself down by straightening the right leg and pressing the left knee to the floor. The left calf is also against the floor, horizontally in front of you. Beware of any pain in the left knee.

With both hands on the floor, lean forward over your left calf, head down and forward. Hold and breathe deeply. Place your elbows and lower arms flat on the floor in front of your left calf and foot.

Let this be a soft pose. Release unnecessary tension in your body and dive into your breath. Direct the breath to the place of sensation, the left hip or inner thigh, which is what you're stretching most. Hold that pose. Often and surrender, release and receive.

Slowly lean back, pulling your left leg back and replacing your left knee to the floor, Push up until you're standing on your knees, spine upright.

Now let's do the same to the other side.

This time, pull the left knee back to a 45-degree angle behind you, pelvis lowered, left leg in front and bent at the knee, foot on the floor. Lean back and inhale while extending your arms to your sides, then bending the elbows to raise the hands upright at the sides of your head. Keep your elbows at a point behind your shoulders.

Set your right hand on the right knee and twist, bringing your left arm across to the right side of your body. Bend the left arm and press the left elbow against the outside of the right knee. Make a fist with your left hand and cover it with your right hand, right elbow up. With the left elbow against the right knee, twist to the right with greater force. Turn your torso up and toward the right. Take a deep breath right in to the belly and then slowly and gracefully release. Don't rush that.

Walk (or inch) your right foot toward the left, then lower yourself down by straightening the left leg and pressing the right knee to the floor. Now your right calf is also against the floor, horizontally in front of you. Again, watch out for any pain in the right knee.

With both hands on the floor, lean forward over your right calf, head down and forward. Hold and breathe deeply. Place your elbows and lower arms flat on the floor in front of your right calf and foot.

Once again, let this be a soft pose. Release unnecessary tension. Direct the breath to the place of sensation, this time the right hip or inner thigh, which is what you're stretching most. Hold that pose. Often and surrender, release and receive.

Now slowly lean back, pulling your left leg back and replacing your left knee to the floor, Push up until you're standing on your knees, spine upright.

Repeat as desired.

Rigorous Option: Yoga Alchemy; The Axis

In this practice we'll look at locating the true center of the being, the essence nature, the divine self. We'll begin with potent core work, vigorous, decidedly physically, to draw attention from the external to the internal; away from turbulent emotion to implacable, incorruptible self.

Start in a downward-facing dog position, with feet and hands on the floor, legs and back straight, pelvis upraised. Raise your right leg up and back and bend at the knee, extending your toes toward the left side of your body. Stretch and hold, breathing deeply. Keep the shoulders square. Keep the left foot strong, the left leg straight and firm. Hold that position and breathe deeply.

Return your right leg to an extended position behind you, straight and strong, before pulling it back in all the way to your chest. Extend your right leg again, back and up and straight. Hold it before bringing it back in to your chest. Repeat this five times, slowly and pausing between positions.

When you bring your right knee in the last time, put your right foot on the floor, keep the left leg extended behind you. Lean back and raise both arms up and back, keeping them straight. Reach upward, stretching your muscles. Hold the position and breathe deeply. Avoid tension in your upper body.

With your hands up, hook your thumbs together and wave your hands and fingers to stretch under-utilized arm muscles. Gently draw your arms back a bit more as you open up your heart center. Release them and let your arms stretch out to the sides to open your chest. Hold and breathe deeply.

Raise your arms to the sky, then bring them together over the heart. Put your hands on the floor and pull both knees in.

Now let's do the same thing to the other side.

Assume the downward-facing dog position, feet and hands on the floor, legs and back straight, pelvis upraised. This time raise your left leg up and back and bend at the knee, extending your toes toward the right side of your body. Stretch and hold, breathing deeply. Keep the shoulders square. Keep the right foot strong, the right leg straight and firm. Hold that position and breathe deeply.

Return your left leg to an extended position behind you, straight and strong, before pulling it back in all the way to your chest. Extend your left leg again, back and up and straight. Hold it before bringing it back in to your chest. Repeat this five times, slowly and pausing between positions.

When you bring your left knee in the last time, put your left foot on the floor, keep the right leg extended behind you. Lean back and raise both arms up and back, keeping them straight. Reach upward, stretching your muscles. Hold the position and breathe deeply. Avoid tension in your upper body.

With your hands up, hook your thumbs together and wave your hands and fingers to stretch under-utilized arm muscles. Gently draw your arms back a bit more as you open up your heart center. Release them and let your arms stretch out to the sides to open your chest. Hold and breathe deeply.

Raise your arms to the sky, then bring them together over the heart. Put your hands on the floor and pull both knees in.

Repeat as desired.

Meditative Option: Meditate with Gratitude

Here one sits to reflect on what one is grateful for; the things which bring joy and calm in a frantic world. You can do this as an option to the other yoga practices, or do it before or afterward or even both.

This is a very simple exercise. Sitting in the lotus position, comfortable with back straight and hands on the knees with palms upturned, simply focus on your breathing as you would in any transcendental meditation session. Feel the breath come in, hold it in the lungs, feel it being expelled in an exhalation. Feel the sensation of the oxygen entering your lungs, your bloodstream, passing through your body.

But with this exercise, once you're relaxed and in tune with your body, focus on slowing down your breath. Do it gradually, and not to extremes.

The idea is to slow the process, to be more mindful, to have more control of the mind over the body, and this is what meditation is all about, especially for our purposes here. You can take as much time as you want, go as slow as you want. But remember to come out of it slowly. Any jarring shift into hyperactivity could be dangerous. Good change is gradual, and a transitional period into and out of this exercise is highly recommended.

Day 3

Gentle Option: Gentle Renewal Flow

This class renews energy, stretches the body, and gently tones muscles. There's a flow from one posture into the next. It includes postures like Warrior 2 and Triangle Pose, then single-leg balancing, along with long holds of hip-opening postures like the Half Pigeon and the Frog/Garland Pose (*Malasana*).

Start with downward facing dog, with feet and hands on the floor, legs straight, hips up and head down. Exhale. Be a step behind your breath, surrender to it. Step your feet to your hands. Rise halfway, gently. Fold deeply, head down and hands on the floor. Inhale as you rise, stretching your arms out at your sides and then up over your head as you stand up straight. Hands together, exhale as you fold forward, bringing your arms in as you lower to the floor, head and hands down (while keeping your legs straight). Raise your left leg in the air as you inhale, lean back and into a lunge position, with your left leg back and straight and your right knee in front of you, right foot on the floor. Lower your right knee to the floor and arch your spine, raising your arms up and back into a crescent moon position.

Twist right and extend your arms to your sides, exhaling. Inhale as you raise your arms upright again and turn to face forward. Hold your left wrist with your right hand and lean to the right while you exhale. Inhale and return to crescent moon position, leaning back with your arms still outstretched above and behind you. Lean forward and return to downward-facing dog.

Now go through it again, this time for the other side.

This time raise your right leg in the hair as you inhale, lean back and into a lunge position, with your right leg back and straight and your left knee in front of you, left foot on the floor. Lower your left knee to the floor and arch your spine, raising your arms up and back into a crescent moon position.

Twist right and extend your arms to your sides, exhaling.

Repeat as desired.

Rigorous Option: Deep, Slow, Mindful Flow

This thorough, full-body class moves at a reasonable pace, but it's still fairly challenging and rigorous. The class seeks to cultivate a balance between ease and effort. It involves twisting and heart-opening balance. Breath is a priority, and the class is suitable for all levels.

Start in a plank position. With fingers and toes on the floor, legs and body straight, hands outside the shoulders. Pull the left leg in so that the outer thigh is against the stomach. Inch the left foot inward so it's to the right of the left hand, but keep the left knee further left of the arm. Your calf should not be in a straight up and down position, but angled so that the knee is projecting to the left. If you think of your leg as two hands on a clock, from your perspective the would read 11:25, not 12:30.

Lean forward just a bit to stretch the muscles and unlock the joints. Now move your left foot to center so that your calf is straight up and down.

Back into a plank position, lower yourself halfway down, inhale and push your head up and back, arching the spine. Take a few deep breaths in this position. Push your toes down and your head back, stretching your core.

Lift your hips and tuck in your head, back into a downward-facing dog position. Lift your heels and stay on your tiptoes as you lean your heels to the right and return them to the floor. Your feet are now horizontal to your body. Feel your beath from your left hand to your left hip joint. Hold that position and breathe deeply. Then shift your heels from the right to the left, keeping your toes firmly fixed on the floor. This time feel the pressure from your right hand to your right hip. Hold and breath before returning to downward-facing dog.

Walk step your feet back to your hands and slowly rise to a standing position.

Repeat as desired.

Meditative Option: Living the Dream; A Vision Meditation

This option has the practitioner looking into the future to envision an ideal condition or situation for their lives. This prepares the mediator for the life they want.

Sitting comfortably (or laying down) and obtaining a calming, regular breathing rhythm, close your eyes and imagine yourself stepping into an elevator. The doors close and you rise; you rise above the worries and complications of your current circumstance. You let go of the pressures and constraints of your present reality. Look up above the doors and see the lights advance, right to left as it takes you higher and further from your anxieties and stresses.

Now the elevator stops and the doors slide open. You are now looking at your idealized life. For you, this is heaven on Earth. What do you see? Is it tropical or mountainous or metropolitan? Where do you live? How is it decorated?

Who's there with you to share it? Where are you? How are you all dressed? There are no constraints, no limits, it's the very maximum of whatever your heart desires. How do you feel?

When you've spent time there, know you'll have to return to your present reality. And transition here is as important as anywhere. Wave goodbye to your family and friends for the time being, knowing you'll see them again soon. Take that elevator back to the ground floor, where you're once again grounded in reality. Your feet may be on the ground, but your head and your heart may remain in the clouds. And isn't that a wonderful thing?

Day 4

Gentle Option: Yin Yoga for Stress Relief

This class offers stress relief through a series of nourishing yin postures which are sequenced so as to unwind your whole being, returning it to a balanced state. The practice will ground you in breath awareness and will take you through a sequence of yin poses to quiets the mind. These postures are carefully chosen to help the joints, relieve lower back pain, and stimulate the parasympathetic nervous system to decrease stress and release anxiety.

This is just one of several stress relief posses which can be held for prolonged periods of time and are great for easing tension. It's the sphynx pose, or the seal pose (they're actually a bit different). Lay flat on the floor, facing downward, with toes extended, elbow and lower arms on the floor in front of you.

For the least amount of back-bend, stack your forearms in front of you with each hand over the opposite elbow. Lower your forehead to rest on your forearms.

For more bending of the spine, pull your elbows back and rest your forearms on the floor in front of you facing either inward with your palms pressed together in the center; or put your arms out straight ahead of you with your palms down. These are variations on the sphynx position. In this position, let your head drop down to stretch the spine and neck and release tension.

Comparable is the seal position, pressing palms flat on the floor in front, straightening the arms and arching the spine, raising the head.

These can all be done with cushions to alleviate soreness and accentuate bending angles more comfortably. Place a yoga cushion under the area of focus and achieve the position. Once there, hold the position and breathe deeply. This position can be held indefinitely, or the cushion can be moved to different spots in rotation.

Rigorous Option: Hatha Yoga; Strength & Freedom

An all-levels Hatha yoga class, this class will tone, warm, and open the body. It's a slow-moving class with long posture holds which strengthen and stretch.

Start with a standing forward bend, legs straight with body bend forward, hands touching the floor. Bow down as deep as your body will allow. Fold inward. Bring your feet together and raise into a chair pose, with knees bent and spine straight but forward-leaning, lifting your arms straight out and up over your head for balance. Reach up as far as you can. Take a deep breath and then, as you exhale, clasp your hands in front of you and bring them to your heart. Lean forward, hands still clasped and knees still bent (even a bit more for balance).

Now twist to the right so that you can place your left elbow outside of your right knee. If you can't do this, put your left hand on the outside of your right knee and place your freed right hand on the small of your back.

Either way, now pull your right shoulder back. Set your hips down a bit and hold this position, breathing deeply. Now go into a forward fold, the position you started with, and do the same for the other side.

Cycle through from the chair position to bringing your hands to your heart. Lean forward, hands still clasped in front of you, knees bent a little more for balance.

Now twist to the left so that you can place your right elbow outside of your left knee. Or put your right hand on the outside of your left knee and place your freed left hand on the small of your back.

Pull your left shoulder back. Set your hips down a bit and hold this position, breathing deeply. Now go into a forward fold, the position you started with, and do the same for the other side.

Repeat as desired.

Meditative Option: Transform Tension to Vitality

This meditation is designed to be done during fasting and during periods of regular diet and weight management. It helps achieve a more restored state to help move the *prana* (life force) through the entire being. This one can be done as an adjunct to another class or on its own.

Sit in a comfortable position, lotus of possible, lying down if necessary. Start with a very deep breath. Now feel your self, your energy, lowering down through your body and into the ground, deep into the Earth. Now feel it coming up again, from the earth and into our body, through your open chest and to the crown of your head. Now exhale, feeling your energy descend back into you and travel downward back to your core. The more you exhale, the further that energy descends. Then inhale again, slowly and naturally, and feel the energy rise. It rises in conjunction with the speed and depth of the breath. The more you inhale the higher it goes, the slower you exhale you lower it descends. This unites the self with the earth below and the sky above, observing the oneness of all thing. But note that you're not controlling the breath, you're simply observing it, understanding it and yourself in a whole new way.

Day 5

Gentle Option: Yin Yoga for Energy and Clarity

Great for a depleted body or spirit, this one is great for when any faster is deep into a fast. This class's yin poses work with the body's chemical intelligence and gently detoxifying the spinal column, kidneys, and enhancing internal organ blood flow.

Begin by lying flat on your back. Pull your right leg up, knee to the chest, placing both hands on the calves just below the knee. Pull gently and breathe deeply. Let your left arm drop down to the floor. Extend your left arm out to your side while your right hand guides your left knee across your body, twisting the lower body to your right. You may have to adjust the angle of your left arm for comfort. Your weight should be on the side of your pelvis with your lower back strong and straight.

Now stretch your right arm out as well, letting your upper body stretch. Now turn your head to the left. Hold and breathe deeply, feel the effects of the twist. Hold this pose as long as you like before returning your head to look directly upward and uncrossing your left leg, once more lying flat with your arms at your sides and your legs together.

Now do the same thing with the other side. Pull your left leg up, knee to the chest, placing both hands on the calves just below the knee. Pull gently and breathe deeply. Let your right arm drop down to the floor. Extend your right arm out to your side while your left hand guides your right knee across your body, twisting the lower body to your left. You may have to adjust the angle of your right arm for comfort.

Now stretch your left arm out as well, then turn your head to the right. Hold and breathe deeply, feel the effects of the twist. Hold this pose as long as you like before returning your head to look directly upward and uncrossing your left leg, once more lying flat with your arms at your sides and your legs together.

Repeat as desired.

Rigorous Option: Earth Yoga

The grounded yoga practice uses gravity to connect the self to its bodily roots and then beyond to its earthly roots. This is a moderately challenging *vinyasa* flow practice which invites balance and stability and which appreciates and honors all the different connections the Earth provides.

Start with downward-facing dog. Walk or hop your feet up to your hands, then halfway lift before going back down in a full forward fold. Rise up straight, arms reaching up, looking up, inhaling. Then exhale as you lower your arms, hands clasped (standing at attention). Release hands and raise them up along the sides and above the head, spine and arms straight.

Follow that up with a forward fold.

Halfway lift, put your hands flat on the floor and walk or hop your feel back, spine and legs straight in a plank position. Press the head back and up, spine arched and arms straight, in a tall cobra position. Inhale then exhale into a downward facing dog.

Inhale and raise the right leg up and back behind you, straight, rotating the right hip to extend the leg as high and straight as possible. Then bend the right leg at the knee, angled toward the left. Hold and breathe deeply. Then straighten the leg, square the hips, and bring the right leg down under the chest, foot on the floor. Extend the left leg, point the left foot outward, and rise up to a standing position with your feet splayed. Extend your arms to your sides, turn your head to look down your right arm to your right hand and beyond. Take your left hand and run it down the left thigh and point the right hand upward. Hold and breathe deeply. Slowly return to a standing at attention position, then lower yourself back into downward dog to repeat for the other side.

Inhale and raise the left leg up and back behind you, straight, rotating the left hip to extend the leg as high and straight as possible. Then bend the left leg at the knee, angled toward the right. Hold and breathe deeply. Then straighten the leg, square the hips, and bring the left leg down under the chest, foot on the floor. Extend the right leg, point the left foot outward, and rise up to a standing position with your feet splayed. Extend your arms to your sides, turn your head to look down your left arm to beyond your left hand. Take your right hand and run it down your right thigh and point the left hand upward. Hold and breathe deeply. Slowly return to a standing at attention position, then lower yourself back into downward dog. Repeat as desired.

Meditative Option: Morning Manifestation Meditation

This short meditation is designed to help energetically and mentally align with your goals for the upcoming day. It should help clear the clutter from your mind and connect to your best intentions and the utmost of your abilities.

Get into a comfortable position, get control of your breathing, locate your energy center and calm it so that it rests peacefully in the core of your being. Now concentrate on what follows; memorize it or have somebody read to you. Read it yourself into a voice recording app on your phone, if that helps. Then let the words pass through you and settle in your brain. Don't fight it; just do it.

Sift through the clutter in your mind. Shelve your to-dos, what's unfinished for now. Sift through the mundane and repetitive thoughts and patterns you may be stuck in so that you can reconnect with your inner intuition, your inner knowing. What emotion is in your space, mind or body or soul, that you don't need, that you want to clear away? Let it go. Acknowledge why it is there, then let it go, especially if it will not serve you today. Allow it to dissolve.

It's easy to imagine your new yoga regiment has you well on your way toward total wellness. You've achieved greater discipline and you've seen and felt the rewards. You're stronger, more capable, more well-informed, more confident. Your body and mind have been more deliberately enjoined and focused to work with one another toward the greater good.

But the journey's not over yet. There are two crucial steps on the journey toward total wellness, greater health and awareness, and master of mind over body. We're reaching the superego promised when the mind/ego controls the body/id. It requires every bit of strength and knowledge this book hopes to offer, and will only encourage both to greater heights. You may already have guessed where we're going, an what we'll be doing next.

Meditation for fasting.

SECTION 7:
MEDITATION FOR FASTING

CHAPTER SIXTEEN: Meditation for Fasting

If you're fasting and dieting and exercising and even doing yoga, you're probably pretty serious about resetting your body and your mind. All of the principles in this book coalesce and intertwine, and they lead us to the world of meditation.

Meditation is an ancient and robust tradition of mental and physical wellness which is derived from the notion that one can separate from one's circumstance, to transcend it, to reach a place of perfect spiritual wholeness.

Like diet, fasting, exercise, and yoga, meditation is easy to lose track of in our cluttered world and amidst our frantic lifestyles. While we're barraged with bad foods, dangerous electronic lighting, long hours and unyielding stress, increased pollutants, desperate economic demands, every opportunity for respite, relaxation, and resetting are robbed from us.

So once again we have to be deliberate and mindful, of what we're doing and how we're living. The paradox is that, while meditation is famous for removing all thought, it is still a mindful practice; more than most, in fact. And while yoga (and fasting) is certainly very deliberate, its goal is to achieve a kind of effortlessness which one can take into other, more challenging facets of modern life.

For this reason, meditation is a solid exercise in discipline. And that discipline is helpful when applied to fasting, exercise, yoga, or any of the things we're discussing in this book. Again, we see how every facet of what we're looking at touches on every facet of everything else. It all connects like some great web of psychological and physiological wellbeing.

Meditation and Weight Loss

Since the body and mind are connected in various ways. And the mind is as powerful a tool as the body. The hand reaches for what the mind allows it to reach for, after all (likely something unconstructive which may please but not benefit and could even harm the body, mind, or soul). And meditation focuses the mind, which makes it a sharp weapon.

Meditation may set the mind free to greater understand the reason the hand reaches for what it wants, the reasons it wants what it wants, reasons the mind does not intervene. When the brain understands what it is doing, it can change the entire chain reaction of behaviors. Meditation allows this the way few things (if anything) can. Along the way, meditation may bring the practitioner closer to core beliefs and childhood disruptions which may be affecting adult behavior. Eating is often a response to stress, anxiety, self-esteem issues, body issues, insecurity, depression, and a host of other destructive conditions and behaviors. Understanding this is the first step toward controlling it. Meditation may be the first step toward greater understanding.

How Meditation Works

For the uninitiated, meditation is grounded in a very simple practice. The idea is to find a relaxed physical condition, either sitting or lying down, standing still or even walking (a more advanced and yet the most pedestrian form of meditation, if you'll pardon the pun). Setting walking aside, imagine sitting still in a quiet place, with your body physically comfortable.

The meditator then chooses one thing to focus on, something very simple. Very often, a beginning meditator begins by focusing on their own breath. This is something which is always accessible to anyone at any time and in any condition. It also connects the meditator to their own body to achieve a kind of closed energy cycle and a stronger connection of body and mind.

The practitioner simply focuses on that single thing, the breath. They focus on the slow inhaling, holding the breath in the lungs, then releasing. The focus isn't on accomplishing the act, which is automatic, but on it is deliberate about breathing; deliberate about intaking the air, holding it for a short but regular count, and deliberate about releasing it. It's about being mindful of how the lungs feel taking in the air, how the blood feels holding it, how the body feels releasing it. It's about focusing on every facet of that often-overlooked but vital practice.

Not everybody chooses their own breath to focus on. Some may choose their own heartbeat, or do a kind of body scan which starts at the feet and guides the focus through every part of the body. Others choose a distant focal point, such as a tree top in the distance, a stain on the wall. Some focus on a monotone they utter, others on a mantra, a repeated phrase. Some focus on envisioning an ideal future for themselves, a perfect mate or house or a family photograph. Some focus on their idea of what God (or a comparable force) might look like.

Some prefer walking as a way of focusing, though there is rarely a single focal point to focus on. This kind of meditation diverts attention to the simple act of walking. Though one isn't so mindful about it as they might be about breathing. Breathing, one concentrates on the inhalation, the exhalation. Though this only lasts a short time, before the mind becomes free of thought as may roam to productive places. When walking, you're not likely to be focusing on the minutia of right foot, left foot. Instead, the focus is drawn by the surroundings, a combination of autonomous movement, breathing, energy management.

Walking is the most popular form of meditation, as people do it so often and it takes little training. People don't think of it as meditating, which is why they do it so often.

Another (but not at all healthy or recommended) type of meditation is the cigarette break. As dangerous and disgusting as this habit is, it does draw the practitioner's attention to breathing, feeling the breath (though chemically charged), savoring the exhalation. Luckily, fewer and fewer people are choosing this type of meditation. It certainly isn't recommended here.

And making that better choice brings us to being deliberate about what we do and how. One may think, for example, that fast food and snack foods are economical. But a USDA study showed recently that $2.50 a day is enough to buy all the natural fruits and vegetables to provide anyone with the recommended weekly caloric allowance.

It's all about being mindful and deliberate, which is what meditating is all about.

Being mindful during a dietary shift like fasting means making and sticking to a new eating plan and having the wisdom and discipline to stick to it. This might entail writing out the weekly menu and putting it on the refrigerator door. Support groups are also often helpful, especially for first-time meditators.

Meditation is Intermittent Fasting for the Mind

We've seen how intermittent fasting can assert mindfulness and deliberateness into our dietary lives, causing autophagy and stimulating the body to reprogram itself. Well, meditation does basically the same thing for the mind.

In fact, the body has two different nervous systems, the autonomic and the voluntary. Automatic behaviors include breathing. Voluntary behaviors include holding your breath. So breath is one of the few places where these two nervous systems meet. This makes it a perfect way achieve a greater connection between body and mind.

In fact, a lot of the potent meditative techniques involve a meeting of these two different aspect of the self, if you will (the automatic and the voluntary). Focal meditation uses the involuntary sense of sight, used in a voluntary way. Hearing is an automatic sense, so hearing your own voice can be said to be a meeting of voluntary and automatic nervous behaviors. Speech is also automatic. Normally, one doesn't have to concentrate on speaking. It's a pity more people don't concentrate on *what* they're saying, but they certainly don't give much thought as to how to say it. How they're saying it is immaterial. But when repeating a mantra, one is deliberate about the pace, the tone, the vibration of the tone in the mouth, the throat, the chest, even resonating throughout the entire body.

And once the body and the mind are more closely connected, the mind has more control over the body and the body less control over the mind. Why is this so? Because the automatic functions have little to do with the mind (but everything to do with the brain). Voluntary functions have everything to do with the brain and the mind. There's much we don't know about the so-called *mind*, so we're in danger of slipping down a rabbit hole here. What we know factually is that a person may be mindfully desirous of moving their hand, but a malfunction of or injury to the brail may prevent it. The brain and the mind are not the same, though they are closely related. And both have sway over the body and can also be swayed by it.

Think of the human being in Freudian terms. Sigmund Freud, the father of modern psychoanalysis, is famous for a number of different contributions to the field. It was Freud who coined the Oedipal and Electra complexes of complex sexual attraction of children to their opposite-gender parents.

Perhaps more famously, Freud has a theory that the human psyche was constructed of three different parts; the ego, the id, and the superego. Freud described the ego as the adult part of the psyche which deals with the outside world; practicality, social behavior. This is the practical adult part of the psyche. The id is the part of the psyche which deals with itself; immediate wants and desires without regard to consequence. This is the child part of the psyche. Freud speculated that every psyche has these two facets inherently. Some people have a stronger ego than others, for some the id is more dominant.

But Freud described a third aspect to the psyche, the superego. This is not inherent, but achieved. The superego is a moral perspective which can only be attained when the practical ego takes and retains control of the childish, selfish id. When the id is dominant, the ego spends all its time satisfying the id and cannot turn its attention to the higher truths and the clarity which is necessary for a strong moral perspective. When the ego controls the id, the superego becomes possible, then and only then.

Now let's think about everything we've looked at in this book so far, the total self. The mind represents the ego, the part of our self which deals with the outside world. It's deliberate, strategic, practical. The body is the id of the whole self, it wants immediate gratification and satisfaction, reaction automatically to stimulus entirely without reason. It reacts with sweat and goosebumps and nausea, hunger and thirst and any number of automatic responses for which it demands satisfaction. Complete wellness (for lack of a better term) is the superego, the moral high ground. It works going backward too; Complete wellness can only be achieved when the practical mind has control over the immaturely selfish body.

You can probably already see where this goes. Everything we've looked at here is about the mind gaining control over the body; fasting, diet, exercise, yoga, understanding hormones and other bodily systems, it's all been about how the mind can control the body.

And meditation is the epitome of the mind controlling the body.

Why is it so important? It brings us back to another phenomenon we've looked at often, and that's the interrelation of systems. One thing influences the other. The mind can control the body and strengthen it by discipline. The body's greater strength inspires the mind to a greater sense of possibility. The mind is rewarded for its efforts toward discipline, and this encourages more discipline, which affects greater strength, which in turn inspires greater discipline.

Let's look at the flipside. When the body gets what it wants all the time, it becomes weak and lethargic, overweight and prone to disease. Disease makes the body weaker. This physical dilapidation affects the mind, which falls into depression from anxiety, stress, and guilt. This generates self-medication (overeating, substance abuses) which further contribute to the maladies which are slowly destroying the body.

In short, these things come in cycles, and one affects the other. The body and mind are inextricably linked. It's only when were mindful of this that we can do something about both. We can see to our bodies through changes in diet and exercise, but meditation is the best way to fine-tune the other major part of the equation; the mind.

Another conundrum about meditation; it's about clearing the mind, but only to allow it to become occupied again. When one focuses on any stimulus, it is not thinking about the chatter of the outside world. It is finding clarity in the jumble of information. But once that clarity is achieved, it remains itself a means to an end. The mind, once cleared, moves on to start thinking about other things, mulling through that chatter and chaos, thinking things through. The clarity is a better way to approach a problem, not a way to avoid or deny it.

Nonjudgmental Awareness

There's an old saying: "All of men's problems arise from his inability to sit quietly for five minutes." This is truer than you may realize. Why? In the day and age people actually used this expression, the 1800s, there was little enough to do and plenty of time to sit quietly. These days, our lives are so hurried and demanding that five quiet minutes actually does seem like a luxury. And with the dominance of electronic entertainment in our culture, five minutes of quiet time is almost unheard of. If we're not letting the TV drone on at home, the internet at work, or our phones while we're on the bus, subway, or plane, we're never without entertainment or input of some kind of content. It's almost as if the powers that be don't want us to be alone with our thoughts. Perhaps they know the great strength there is to it, and how much of a manipulative hold they'd lose over such a huge buying audience.

Either way, finding five minutes to sit alone isn't as easy or as common as you might think.; unless you're mindful and deliberate about it. You might set a certain time aside every day, first thing in the morning or last thing before bed or tea time at four in the afternoon. You may do it opportunistically, when the moment arises. But it's important to do it.

Think of it as nonjudgmental awareness.

The key to it is that it's not really meditating in that it doesn't require a focus on a single focal point or bodily system or mantra. This is the kind of meditating one does on a walk. Instead of thinking precisely about one thing, one thinks basically of nothing. The same kind of clarity is still achieved, and it is automated in a certain sense. If you're sitting or walking or taking a shower, you're still engaged in a cluster of automatic behaviors, though when they're combined they're just a bit more deliberate.

If you're sitting looking out the window, don't think about trimming the trees or anything too deliberate. Just sit and stare. There are no answers on that tree, the answer is in the looking.

This is actually a common trick among various professionals, including those who have to puzzle over tricky concepts or principles. These can be lawyers circling around a tricky problem for their client, writers working out story questions, social workers and doctors and all manner of professionals. When one concentrates too much on a problem, a forest-for-the-tress problem sets in. Overthinking a problem can jam up the rational system. So stepping away from the problem to perform some perfunctory physical chore is a good way to distract the mind just enough. This is often called *thought showering* because taking a shower requires a group of fairly automatic but still voluntary actions which require just enough conscious though to distract the mind. This often frees up the mental jam and lets an answer become easy to find. Walking is a popular way to implement the same method of bringing body and mind together and letting one influence the other in a positive, deliberate fashion.

Another aspect to nonjudgmental awareness is actually about not judging what you see. It's more than just not being distracted by your tree branches, but your neighbor's yard. It's hard to be aware and not be judgmental. We're trained from childhood to have cognitive and critical thinking skills, and this requires a certain amount of information processing and problem solving. The problems are that (firstly) people are not problems, they *have* problems which can be solved; and (secondly) children are not equipped to understand the subtleties between understanding things and judging them. They're often never taught these differences, as often enough their parents don't know the differences either. It's another subject for another book, one of several on the subject from our own library perhaps. But for our purposes here, there is a difference between a person and their actions, opinions, mistakes. The clear mind will see this, and meditation will make that clear.

Transcendental Meditation

Here is the meditation we've all come to know, sitting quietly focusing on the breath, a focal point, a mantra. It's about stillness and quiet, focusing concertedly on one thing to the exclusion of everything else. It's great for clarity, for mental sharpness, for discipline in every way.

When thoughts do appear in the uncluttered mind, they are easier to understand, and so the answers are easier to see. This practice may be done for five minutes a day for clarity management, or for an hour or several hours at a time.

An hour a day is recommended for serious meditation. It's as good a way to spend an hour at night as, say, watching reruns of *South Park* or *Peep Show*. And the more you watch the news, the more the calming effects of meditation may be helpful and even required. So for that one hour, don't be fearful. We spend so much of our lives in fear. Our bodies and minds are guided by a fight-or-flight response, which is basically fear incarnate. Our society teaches us to be fearful of just about everything; strangers, social scorn, sexually transmitted disease, gun violence, terrorism.

But for an hour a day of meditation, give up the fear, transcend it. Focus on your selected point of interest; your breath, your mantra, your body, your stained wall. Let go of everything else, especially the fear.

There's also a matter of guilt. Because our lives are so demanding, because time is so short, it may be hard to justify taking an entire hour to do absolutely nothing. But we know meditating is so much more than nothing, it only appears to be that. The benefits are almost unending and are plain to see even in a short dissertation like this one. But it's easy to allow the pressures of life to infiltrate on that hour of meditation, even to prevent it. So it takes discipline and resolve to declare one's own right to this kind of selfcare. Don't be afraid, and don't be guilty, just do it.

Once you've let go of the guilts and the fears of the present, you can begin to let go of the fears of the past. Meditation of this quantity and quality will allow reflection and introspection to allow one to transcend emotional corruption and chaos and discover rational and reasonable clarity. Then you can rationally overcome those lingering pains and negative feelings which cause so much present-day misbehavior and self-sabotage.

Meditation is the best way to make those old, lingering pains clear and to exorcise them. It's a mental kind of autophagy, and it's even more beneficial to overall good health.

Along those lines, be nonjudgmental about the thoughts which your new clarity brings you to. Don't fight them or deny them or blot them out. If they face you, face them back. This is what meditation is basically for, after all. You have nothing to be fearful of nor guilty over.

It isn't always easy or convenient, but what is easy and convenient is also often harmful to us, body and mind, as we have seen. Be deliberate and mindful, use the discipline of the ego to control the immature id of your body. Achieve the superego's superior vision of better greater wellness.

All this meditation will bring you more closely in tune with psyche, your ego with your id. You'll learn to recognize how your mind and body may be disjointed and help you on the long road to reunion of the two. It won't happen overnight. Good change is gradual change.

But once you recognize your lesser self, once your mind has achieved control over your body (instead of the other way around), you'll be able to exercise that control with greater deliberation.

Before we move on to the specialized program we've arranged, let's take a quick look at some meditation apps, some of which will likely prove helpful to you in your quest for total wellness via intermittent fasting. Note: Some of these are free, others offer subscription add-ons. We suggest you double-check their prices, as these are subject to change.

Meditation Apps

Calm is considered the best of the best among experts. The app's guided meditations do more than lead you through anxiety and lack of focus, but they do a lot more than that! These benefits include:
- Different tools and modalities
- Well-being offerings such as sleep stories
- Celebrity voicings (including Matthew McConaughey)

Insight Timer offers features few others can match, including:
- Over 45K free meditations
- Filtering by need or goal, duration, or benefit
- Seven-day free trial/meditation introductory course
- Supportive community

Headspace Meditation & Sleep is popular for those trying to get to sleep, often a problem during a fast. It offers:
- Breathing exercises

- Wind-down practices
- sleep meditations
- dim, meditation-friendly lighting

Ten Percent Happier Meditation is based on the popular book. It's a good way to mainstream the meditation experience. It offers:

- Short, on-the-go sessions
- Mindful day tracking

Unplug is handy for those with little time to meditate. Even five minutes is enough to unplug with this popular app, which offers:

- User self-direction
- Ambient sounds and timers
- Ideal for refocus during stress
- 30-day challenge

Habit is perhaps the best for simple use. Modern users are often looking for more simplicity in their lives, not more complexity. So this app may be the best choice, offering:

- Quick, on-the-go meditation
- Extensive meditations library
- Clearly organized

- Special meditations to lessen stress and combat panic attacks
- Offline use (with premium subscription)

And now, as we did before, we'll apply all this new knowledge to some real-time physical applications. We've fasted, we've dieted, we've exercised, we've done some yoga. Now it's time to meditate. Of everything we've looked at, meditation may be the most user-friendly and the most beneficial. It certainly will tie all of your previous practices together.

CHAPTER SEVENTEEN: Meditation Programs for Fasting and the Immunity System

Meditation Program for Fasting

The purpose of this meditation is to guide your mind towards better health. Before we begin, find a comfortable position, either on the floor, in a chair, or on a bed. Let your back be straight and upright. Remain present and open minded. Close your eyes and take a long, slow breath in through the nose. Breathe in and out, long and slow, a few more times. The longer and the slower, the better.

Your mind is clear. Your awareness is here. You feel safe and relaxed while engaged in this meditation. When I talk about self, when you think about self, we focus on the awareness which is currently taking in these words, hearing them and feeling them resonate through the entire body.

If you're fasting, you are already healing your body and mind. You are extending your lifespan and improving the later years of your life. Imagine a life which becomes more enjoyable as we age. Obesity, heart issues, cancer, it's a long lit of ailments which fasting can prevent. Eating only when we are truly hungry creates the utmost self-respect. The idea of eating multiple small meals per day does not give the body time to begin the healing process. This process is vital to clean out the body's impurities. Abstinence of food gives us a new, sharpened mental discipline which converts itself into a force of freedom. By freedom, we mean freedom within your mental or physical health. Fasting and eating appropriately will provide extra vitality, and that is the essence of life. Now you can spend more time with family as a more energized, healthier individual who leads life to the fullest.

Relax your body and mind now, knowing that you are already well onward in your journey.

Feel what is through your senses. Understand that you are not your senses, you are only using them to observe yourself and your reality. Meditate. Listen to whatever sound there is in the room, even if that's only vague sounds leaking in from the outside.

Now take a deep breath in through the nose and let it out through the mouth. Do that again. You are fasting again, getting healthier with every passing minute. You mut keep the regime up, even though it will at times be difficult. The rewards are worth the effort. It's too important for you not to give up, however difficult it may be.

Visualize yourself living the best life possible, free of disease, high in energy and appreciation. Visualize yourself sharing it with those you know and love. Fasting will bring that reality to you, so let it guide you toward that ideal future and let that ideal future guide you through your fasting regiment.

Return your awareness slowly to the room, to your body. Center on your heart and then slowly bring your awareness outward to the rest of your body. Shrug your shoulders as you feel that energy pass outward through them. Bend your spine slowly from side to side, muscles gently pushing at the vertebrae to release excess tension.

Meditation Program for the Immune System

The purpose of this meditation is to improve your immune system through self-reflection and meditation. These are easy and effective ideas which may help you improve our immune system.

Allow yourself to be comfortable, but not too comfortable. You should be sitting up, with back straight, leaning on some pillows. Roll your head a few times to loosen your neck so you can be relaxed and focused.

Connect to the breath by inhaling through the nose and exhaling through the mouth, slowly and deliberately. Do this repeatedly until your body and mind are in a tranquil, open state. Bring your awareness into the center of your mind. Greet it, come to know it. Slow it down and connect with your immune system. Focus on connecting to the white blood cells, which govern your immune system.

Greet them. Note how you feel when you familiarize yourself with the immune system.

Even considering the immune system makes it stronger, by focusing the body's attention on it. And considering it is a form of meditation. You're already on your journey toward tranquility and away from stress, getting further along with every breath in through the nose, every moment holding it, and every moment during the exhalation.

Begin concentrating on your feet. Feel your toes, move them around and flex them. Sense the bones, the tendons. Then move up to the feet, arch and twist them, roll them on your ankles. Then focus on your calves, the muscles pulling and contracting and releasing at your whim. Get a sense of the skin stretched over that muscle, the hair on that skin if there is any. Then move your attention upward. Feel your thighs, the strong femur bone, the tendons stretching from the knees to the hips. Feel your groin, the center of the body. Be aware of it, the physical and mystical power of the genitals, the base of the vital organs as you feel your way through your own digestive tract. Sense the congestion if there is any.

Remember to be breathing deeply but steadily as you do this meditative survey. Keep scanning up to your stomach, your kidneys and liver, your spine. Be mindful of every part of your body, what its function is and what its condition is. Be even more mindful of your breathing as your scan takes you to the lungs, expanding and contracting, your heart beating steadily. Is the heartbeat steady? Keep it calm without having to wrestle control over it. Work with it, not against it. Be aware of your bones, ribs strong and protective.

Feel your shoulders, is the tension still there from before? Scan down the length of your arms, down the muscles to the elbows, down the forearm to the wrist and hand, where tiny bones intermingle with tendons, nerves, and muscles in a most delicate way. Think about those frail bones which do so much work, so much of the time. Feel your nerves and tendons and bones right to the tips of your fingernails.

Now come back, revisiting the arms on your way back to the shoulders, the neck, the spine in this delicate area. Scan your head, your jaw and teeth, your ears and face, your nose and eyes. Bring your focus right up to the top of your head, completing the full meditative scan.

Now do it again, but this time you'll have some familiarity with how each part of your body feels. Start at the head and work your way down, revisiting areas which you'd overlooked for so long. It's on this second scan that things become more noticeable; little pangs or pains, twitches or stiffness or weakness now become more apparent. It's like re-reading something for errors. The more often you read it, the more errors you notice ... and can correct.

Once you have scanned your body twice, pull back and see it as if for the first time. What does it look like, what does it smell like? Is it in its prime, or in clear decline? Make sure your body is as aware of it as you may now be, and direct your body's resources to those areas both with your body (physical exercises and yoga positions) and your mind (meditation, discipline).

Envision that future version of yourself and your life, as you did before. What does that you look like? What diseases have been rid of that version of you? Let those visions replace doubt anxiety and doubt.

Imagine yourself transforming into that person, becoming them with every breath, with every new or newly repaired cell, with every better dietary choice you make, with every walk you take.

Early morning walks and late-night bike rides are pleasant ways to exercise the body we currently inhabit. We must be mindful not to overstress it, to let its healthy functions take place. Daily exercise is crucial to a healthy lifestyle. There are no short cuts, no magic pills. A healthy body is a mindset, and a mindset is a state of mind. A state of mind is an awareness, and this is an awareness of who we are and who we could be; living a strong, peaceful, contented life with everything we want in life.

Take another deep breath in through the nose to focus on awareness before releasing a big sigh of awareness. We're focusing on making better decisions in our lives, and our immune systems will function better as a result. The exercises don't have to be strenuous, and heathy food tastes delicious. It makes us feel energized toward life, so we can live longer and appreciate the quality of life. It allows us to focus our attention on our internal heat. Heat fosters relaxation. Picture a sauna, relaxing the body, detoxifying through sweating, allowing autophagy and rebirth throughout the body.

Take another deep breath and bring your awareness back to your shoulders. Roll your head again on your shoulders as you did at the beginning of the meditation to bring your awareness back to your body, to remain loose going into the rest of the day.

One might think we've gone as far into the mind as we can, and in a way our journey has indeed gone from the physical (fasting, dieting, exercising) to the mental (yoga, meditation). But there's one step further to go, one which transcends both body and mind and yet draws them together in a way that nothing else can. It is neither nutritional nor dietary, nor is it recognized as an aspect of mental health or even psychology or psychiatry. It is the last frontier of non-traditional treatment which has already demonstrated a history of efficacy in a variety of ways. There things it can't cure and things it can. Once you come to know it better, to master it, you'll know if it can save your life or merely improve it. Prepare yourself, as you're about to go to the final step in our journey toward the ultimate reunion of body and mind, total wellness.

Hypnotism.

SECTION 8: HYPNOTISM

CHAPTER EIGHTEEN: Hypno-fasting

Hypno-fasting may sound like a new approach, and it may be, depending on how you look at it. Hypnosis itself is fairly new to the human experience, and there's a lot we still don't know or understand about it. But the link between hypnosis and weight loss is longstanding and well-established. As soon as people recognized hypnosis as a remedy, weight loss was one of the first maladies they turned it to. And that only makes sense. Both are often misunderstood, and weight loss has been such a stubborn (and increasingly threatening) problem that it only makes sense that seemingly drastic measures such as hypnosis would soon be taken. This was when diet and weight loss were not so well understood as they are today. Even so, hypnosis had proven a potent remedy for any number of things, for reasons still now quite known. It's too functional and effective to simply discount. And with our opened minds and opened hearts, with our greater understanding of physiological actions and reactions, its time to turn our attention to this final frontier of overall wellness.

Hypnosis.

History

As much of a post-psychoanalytic novelty as it might seem, hypnosis actually dates all the way back to the ancient empires Greece and Egypt. The word *hypnos* refers to a Greek God of the same name, and it is the Greek word meaning *sleep*. Keep in mind here that, though considered ancient and, by some, primitive, each of these bygone empires accomplished feats of engineering with the minimal tools of the age which today's modern computer technology could not hope to replicate. So consider the geometric perfection of the Pyramids of Giza or the deliberate imperfection of the Parthenon atop the Acropolis in Athens. (For those who don't know, the seemingly perfect geometry of the building is an illusion, using forced perspective to give the illusion of geometric perfection. In truth the building is riddled with deliberately inaccurate angles which will look perfect from afar.)

So if these cultures (which also pioneered brain surgery) took hypnosis seriously, perhaps we should too.

Both the Greek and Egyptian cultures had religious centers where people sought consultation. Hypnosis of a sort was used to induce and interpret dreams, to envision oracles. Ancient writings are replete with references of the sort. Indeed, most of John of Patmos' Book of Revelation is said to have been written in an hypnotic, trance-like state.

In 2600 BC Wong Tai, the father of Chinese medicine, recorded techniques involving incantations. In 1500, BC, the Hindu Vedas chronicled techniques involving certain hypnotic procedures. Druidic, shamanistic, yogic, voodoo, and other religious practices rely on a trance-like state induced by some form of hypnotism.

Franz Mesmer (1734 – 1815) is said to be the father of modern hypnosis. The word *mesmerize* is derived from his name. He was maligned in his time (and often enough, today) but he was a pioneer and a genius. He was the man who developed the now-accepted theory of animal magnetism, which states that diseases are resultant from blockages of magnetic forces inside the body.

Mesmer became popular defining the image of a hypnotist; goatee, black cape, magnetic eyes. He was rebellious and theatrical, and we wouldn't have hypnosis (as we know it) without him.

London University professor John Elliotson (1791 – 1868), who introducied the stethoscope to England, was forced to resign after championing the use of mesmerism (soon to be called *hypnosis*). He went on to give numerous private demonstrations, furthering the increasing interest and literature on the little-understood subject.

Mid-nineteenth-century Britain James Braid (1795 – 1860) was a Scottish eye doctor when he found a patient staring into a lamp, seemingly dazed.

He was responsive to Braid's commands, sparking Braid's interest in the field. Getting a patient to fixate on a certain thing (as one does in transcendental meditation) was a critical aspect of hypnotism. A swinging watch, a swirling disk, even the hypnotist's fingertips or eyes, are popular focal points to use during hypnosis. Braid's work remains a cornerstone for contemporary studies on the subject.

British surgeon James Esdaile (1808 – 1859) saw the potency of hypnosis on pain relief and actually performed many hundreds of major surgical operations using only hypnotism as an anesthetic.

Frenchmen J.M. Charcot (1825 – 1893), Ambrose Liébeault (1823 – 1904), and Charles Richet (1850 – 1935) also did impressive work furthering the art and craft of hypnosis. Emile Coué (1857 – 1926) pioneered auto-suggestion. He coined the phrase made popular in The Beatles' song, *Getting' Better*: "Day by day in every way I am getting better and better." He believed in guiding people toward self-healing, which is where hypnosis begins to work its way into our current field of concern. He believed, in fact, that there was no such thing as hypnosis, only self-hypnosis.

In a sense Coué also anticipated the placebo effect – treatment of no intrinsic value the power of which lies in suggestion: patients are told that they are being given a drug that will cure them. Recent research on placebos is quite startling. In some cases statistics indicate that placebos can work better than many of modern medicine's most popular drugs. It seems that while drugs are not always necessary for recovery from illness belief in recovery is!

Even Sigmund Freud (1856 – 1939) showed an interested in the advancing field of hypnosis, but his work took into the area of psychoanalysis, for which he became famous. For Freud, remedy was not found by the patient alone, but through careful guidance by a trained professional.

In the modern era, Milton H. Erickson, MD (1901-1980), advanced hypnosis after suffering with polio-induced paralysis as a child. It gave him a window into human psychology. Erickson's work remains the most popularly cited in the study and application of hypnosis today and his techniques are considered the most effective.

Experts now are more ready to accept the connection of hypnosis and medicine.

What is Hypno-fasting?

Hypno-fasting combines intermittent fasting with various techniques of hypnotherapy/hypnosis toward the specific goal of losing weight through fasting.

Intermittent fasting is proven to have beneficial effects, that's true. But it can be difficult for some people. We're trained throughout our lives to rely on three meals a day, and those meals get bigger and bigger while offering fewer nutrients. Psychologically, physically, and socially, we've become addicted to the habitual act of eating, regardless of nutritional necessity. It's more than just temptation for satisfaction, it's a matter of a lifetime of training. It can be hard to reverse such deeply engrained patterns.

Hypnosis can help with that, because habits are practiced in the body, but they're born of the mind. Once you've been through the practices in this book, your mind will be stronger, its relationship to our body should be more dominant. If so, that'll help with hypnosis during your fasts. If not, hypnosis will help you achieve that mental mastery.

Hypnotism as useful on the young as the old, and it works regardless of health, wealth, race, creed, or social strata. Rich or poor, fat or thin, hypnosis has no differential of efficacy.

Hypnosis is not mind-control or magic. A person cannot really be made to do something they do not want to do (sorry, fans of *The Manchurian Candidate*). Hypnotic blackouts are also mythological, as is the idea of being stuck in hypnosis and never snapping back to reality. Really, minor states of hypnosis happen all the time without any theatrics or swinging watches on gold chains. It may happen to you every time your mind just wanders, every time you lose yourself in thought. It may happen several times a day, depending on who you are, where you are, and what your mind is normally like.

Hypnosis is, like other things we've studied, a way to direct focus in order to block out other distractions, the basic principle of meditation. And, as with meditation, it's a conscious state, not a zombie-like sleepwalking state of perfect suggestibility. Those who have been hypnotized describe is as the feeling one has just as they fall asleep; awake, but so relaxed that even movement seems unnecessary.

Experts agree that nobody is truly beyond hypnotism. Some are more open to it, more responsive, some will naturally be more closed and more resistant. One thing is for sure; if you don't want to be hypnotized, you won't be. The subject (for lack of a better word) plays an active part in the process, and that requires an open heart and an open mind.

And, like intermittent fasting, this kind of hypnosis, hypno-fasting, can be sustained for an indeterminant amount of time; regularly for the rest of your life, if you like. You're developing parallel skills of self-discipline and self-awareness. Both are excellent for tightening your focus, and that will help you in other endeavors. The more you do both, the better you'll get at them, and at related practices as we've gone over here. Your exercising regiment should be accented by the discipline you've learned and earned during a fast, and that energy will transfer to the self-awareness you achieve during yoga and meditation.

Hypnosis will not eradicate the hunger a fast brings on, that will come and go. But it will help you accept it instead of fighting against it. It will help you embrace that hunger as a necessary part of your life and as a necessary part of your growth.

Hypnosis Apps

We'll be going through some actual hypno-fasting courses soon, when you'll be able to put this fascinating concept into practice. But first, let's take a look at one of the newest revolutions in hypnosis, the hypnosis app.

This should come as a surprise to nobody. They have apps for everything, after all. We've already taken a look at apps for yoga and for exercise and even for fasting. And hypnosis is an ideal way to partake of this kind of practice without disrupting anybody else's schedule.

Some people don't like apps, or don't have app-worthy phones. Others prefer the company of others. Either way, there are apps for that, and here are the best ones:

Hypnobox is regarded by many as the best self-hypnosis app. It's designed to achieve a state of deep relaxation. This leans on the notion that being in a highly relaxed state makes one more open to suggestions of new behaviors and thoughts. The app can be customized with a male or female voice, and you can tailor your sessions and import your own background music.

Relax and Sleep Well Hypnosis focuses on techniques for relaxation and offers sessions on stress, anxiety, self-esteem, and mindfulness.

Harmony Hypnosis Meditation offers music, mantras, visual images, even sound effects.

Perhaps the best one for losing weight is the aptly named Lose Weight Hypnosis app. The app's audio sessions utilize suggestions to influence behavior and mindset subconsciously. User reviews suggest the app is useful for weight loss and relaxation both.

Digipill is well-known for relieving stress. It's also a well-known health and fitness app which uses psychoacoustics and the hypnosis style known as *neurolinguistic programming.* Psychoacoustics uses sound to induce psychological response. It's a type of neurolinguistic programming, which postulates a strong connection between sensory experiences, behaviors, and emotions. The app offers different programs for weight loss, stress relief, weight loss, motivation, and smoking cessation.

Anxiety Free's app seeks to relieve anxiety via self-hypnosis and guides users through activities meant to relieve stress. One study suggests self-hypnosis may be effective for ongoing anxiety and for situational anxiety, which occurs from a specific past, present, or future event.

Now let's get to it, shall we? You're probably already experienced in at least one or two of the practices in this book, though not necessarily. Don't feel bad if you haven't lifted a single knee. Feel free to read through these hypnosis programs first. You may be recording them on a voice recorder app, after all. But reading the material through first will let it sink in on one level before saying it helps the material sink in even deeper. Listening to it will give you a third listen in your first session, and that can only improve its efficacy. Repetition is what this kind of hypno-fasting is all about.

CHAPTER NINETEEN: Hypnosis Programs

Now we present six one-hour hypnosis programs, one each for the things we've been discussing: Fasting, weight loss, food addiction, emotional eating, body anxiety, and sleep.

Some necessary notes here: These programs are meant to be spoken. Using whatever devices you used before, either pre-recording or using a partner, there are some things to keep in mind.

Read the text slowly. It is not meant to be rushed through, but to be languid and deliberate and mindful. The words have meaning, even the sounds of the words have meaning. When reading them, let the words linger on the tongue, let the speaker by mindful of their importance, of their rhythm.

Create a soothing tone with the text. Speak in a low tone, soft, not sharp or shrill. Imbue the reading with the nurturing and supportive spirit of the sessions. Whether or not you are prerecording the scripts, you may want to include background music, of course of a soothing nature. Sound effects may be appropriate too, including the sounds of wind, rain, birds singing, a babbling brook, whatever seems or feels appropriate. These programs are meant to help you, so you should have a say in how they sound. It could make all the difference in how they affect you.

True, reading them into a voice recorder app may not give you much creative flexibility, but you can always read the script into a a laptop with Garage Band or a comparable recording program and you can easily download and add whatever music or sound effects that you like. You can record and add your own music if you like.

If you have a partner reading the scripts, you can find plenty of sources of ambient sounds and music that are perfect for this practice. However you do it, there's no reason not to begin. You have nothing but choices and a beautiful, ideal future waiting ahead.

We'll begin with hypno-fasting and proceed from there. We do suggest you not skip ahead. Like the rest of this book, these are carefully sequenced to build one upon the other. Trust us, we know what we're doing.

Hypno-fasting

Fasting may help to improve the natural functioning of your brain. It may make you realize (and this escapes a lot of people) that you are only a humble human being. As your body's stored toxins are released, you will feel refreshed and ready to take on all the challenges that life has to offer.

Some doctors believe that pure water fasting may do more than detoxify cells and rejuvenate organs. It may actually cure some diseases. They believe fasting is nature's natural restoration mechanism.

Whyever you have decided to fast, you are going to use your creative subconscious mind to help you to maintain your resolve and to make fasting a pleasant, rewarding, and even an easy experience.

Visualization is the domain of the brain, its native language. In a moment, I will ask you to envision certain things. And I will ask you to envision the scenes as I describe them to you; envision them to the best of your ability.

Perceive any smells or sounds that accompany these impressions. You will find that, in envisioning the scenes, you may go further, deeper into a gentle hypnotic rest.

And with each of your breaths and each of my words, you will be drifting deeper into a calm. Your body becomes more at rest, more at ease. Your troubles are all faded and forgotten, your mind is at peace. Your heart is beating evenly, untroubled. Your blood moves easily in your veins, smoothly, your skin and your muscles feel relaxed.

You take a deep breath and hold it, let it refresh and relax you. Now release the breath again, feeling your chest going down as the air goes out, taking with it any trace of discomfort, any shadow of doubt. You have no preconceptions, you have no desires, you have no thoughts at all. You are loose, you are relaxed, your mind and body are at one and both are perfectly at ease as you listen to the sound of my voice. Your mind is receptive, your heart is open. You are ready for where you are about to go and what you are about to do. Your subconscious mind is set to go, there is nothing holding it back. There is nothing holding you back.

Envision yourself in your home. But this is not the apartment or house you live in. It is the room in your brain where your thoughts are stored.

You are surrounded by shelves of books, papers, and objects; all shapes and sorts and sizes. The books and papers cover a wide variety of subjects. Some of the books are old and others are new.

All the items on the shelves represent things you think about often.

There sits some paperwork relating to your job, piles of bills, photos of your friends and family, souvenirs from your vacation, items to represent your hobbies and interests and various other things. You are starting to fast, or you are about to begin fasting. Food is on your mind. But in order to help you succeed in your fasting, thoughts of food must be shunted, put aside.

One wall of the room has numerous cupboards, and a refrigerator and freezer.

Walk over to it. The cupboards are filled with the thoughts of all your favorite foods. You gather a few large empty cardboard boxes and begin filling them with everything to do with food.

The cupboards are bare; your mind has been emptied of all thoughts of food. You are left with filled-up boxes that you drag outside, ready to be carted off.

Go back inside, admire your accomplishment. Survey all the clean empty shelves. You have done something significant here, and you feel lighter inside, clean just as the cupboards are clean. You cannot quite remember what was on them, it does not matter. There are always new thoughts in your mind that need a shelf. And the new things you will store there will be better, fresher, made for new life and better times. They will be the memories of the better choices you make now, the better things you are now better able to do.

Since the shelves are empty and you have cleared the clutter, you may now move ahead with you fasting amid fewer distractions. Your mind is clear and your thoughts are positive. You enjoy detoxifying your body. It is an added bonus, but also crucial, to detoxify your mind. Fasting may help improve your mental clarity, concentration, and focus. It is a transformative practice for a better, more spiritual life.

You may not see a spiritual star in your life, but that does not mean there isn't one there. It could mean that you hasn't found it yet. Or, like all stars, it could be travelling light years across space and time to reach you, and it may not have appeared in your life's sky as yet. That does not mean that it is not there.

But you have nothing to fear either way. You are your own source of strength, your own star. You do not need a higher power, you already have access to a higher power within you. You are a higher power. All you have to do is look within to see everything that is without. That power allows you to go anywhere, see anything, do anything, even fasting.

Fasting requires self-discipline. This gives you a feeling of being in greater control of your life. It increases your confidence in the choices you make. It fills you with a new and yet familiar strength. It is the strength of the best you, the alpha you. This is the person you were designed to be, the person you were meant to be. Enjoy the feeling of that strength, in your blood, in your muscles. You are strong and you are getting stronger. Feel that strength increasing with every breath, gathering up to face any challenge, withstand any storm.

You recognize that your system does not need (nor does it want) to be overloaded with food. You enjoy a new feeling of lightness in your body and mind. Your blood insulin, sugar, and cholesterol levels are in balance. Your metabolism and fat-burning systems are slowly strengthening. Every part of your body, every cell, is working toward your optimal health. The body is healing and caring for itself because you are allowing it to. You are our own champion, and you are standing up for yourself at long last.

And you are fighting a grievous enemy; illusion. Illusion is at the heart of so much of what we're combating together on your journey to total wellness. It is illusion which manipulates our self-images. It is illusion which makes us think we will be satisfied by processed, fried foods. It is illusion which prevents us from investigating paths to truer consciousness, like yoga and meditation. This entire book is a rally against the illusions which are preventing you from achieving, from loving and doing, from living and from being.

Now you have the truth, which vanquishes illusion. Now you have the power to cast aside old pains which you believe still have power over you. But those things are gone, and their influence over you is the influence of an illusion. Now you are armed with the tools you need, the truth, to remove illusion as a road block on your journey to total wellness. It has held you back for too long, blocked your way and kept you from getting ahead.

But no more.

Even now, the changes are underway. Even now autophagy is replenishing your cellular supply. This very instant, your body is detoxifying, clearing away the old to make way for the new. This is a moment of revelation for you, body and mind. All the cellular changes are happening inside your body. Your body is cleansing and repairing itself. You feel an inner sense of peace, calm, and tranquility. Any problems that you have previously experienced in your life fade away. They become insignificant and you become connected to the higher forces around you.

Recognize this as an entity which you are comprised of; flesh and spirit. When you give your physical self the rest it craves, this allows the spiritual side of you to grow and refine. As it grows, you become more aware of your place in the Universe. Your relationship to others and the importance of love and kindness changes.

You enjoy fasting and savor the inner sense of satisfaction which may never be provided by food. You may decide to fast intermittently to encourage healing and transformation and promote peace and harmony at the very deepest level of your body-mind system. Visualize yourself going through a day of fasting in a calm and peaceful way.

Envision that you are starting to feel a bit hungry. Envision a balloon and place it in your stomach, right where the hunger was. Once your balloon is in place, you can pump it up by taking a sip of water. If water is not allowed, swallow your saliva.

The water travels to your stomach and inflates that balloon, relieving your stomach of its hungry feeling. It fills you. It leaves no room for anything else. It occupies your empty places. You are full, you have no need for more food. Your body craves fasting, it denies food. It knows that food would interrupt the good work it is doing. Your body is grateful for what you are doing for it, for allowing it to repair itself.

And you are glad to be able to help. You and your body have a healthier relationship now, a stronger alliance. You are its champion.

Look around the room. Look at the shelves which you cleared. If any thoughts of food have returned to the shelves, you clear them off once again and place them into another empty box, ready for disposal.

The suggestions are embedded in your subconscious mind. They grow stronger every day. You can fast whenever you wish to with complete willpower. You will know that no negative thoughts of hunger or food will be able to stand in your way.

And this will happen; not just because I say so, but because you have decided it will. That is correct; you have decided, you and your subconscious mind.

Trust yourself. You know by instinct when it is time to fast and when it is time to break that fast. When it is time to continue eating again, you will know the time is right. You eat healthier than ever, and you feel better each time.

You know the importance of maintaining a healthy diet and you know when it is time to have a rest from eating and give your body and mind time to repair. And fasting is easier for you and you enjoy it. You take satisfaction from being able to demonstrate your power of mental determination to yourself and to the world.

I'm going to count the numbers from one to five. At the count of five, you will be wide awake, fully alert, refreshed and ready to allow the suggestions to work for you. And the suggestions will grow stronger by the day, stronger by the hour, stronger by the minute.

Prepare yourself as I count up to five. You will come all the way back to me at the count of five.

One, two, three … begin coming back. Four … your eyelids are starting to flutter. And … five. Your eyes are opening, your mind and body are returning to your full conscious awareness. You feel alert and refreshed and ready to commence your period of fast.

End session.

Relax and reflect. Breathe deeply, give yourself some time to transmission out of your state and back to a grounded, healthy perspective. How do you feel after your first session? What did you learn about your powers to envision? Did you build on the visionary skills and abilities you developed earlier, in your meditations? Did you find solace in what you envisioned? How did you feel at the end of the session?

How does it make you feel during your fasting? Did you pick up some useful tools to get you through the more challenging aspects of the fast? Could you feel that balloon in your belly, pushing away any room for food? Did you sense the control of your mind over your body? Do you sense it?

Remember as you go on with your fasting that you are always in control. If you use these hypnotic techniques or if the other techniques in this book are going to be enough will be up to you. But even more important than any constructive tools you take away is the overall feeling you have as a result of the experiment. Savor the calm, the sense of unity with yourself. You have seen yourself in a new light, and you should be imbued with a new confidence, a sense that you have insight which others do not have.

And you have gained some invaluable experience just by participating in the exercise. Your question about hypnotism have been answered, your doubts have been allayed. You are not clucking like a chicken, right? You are not walking around like a zombie, bumping into walls. you know how it feels, you know what to expect. And you are ready to move on to the next program. From fasting, we move to weight loss, and then onward!

Weight Loss

Feel relaxed and at ease, your body loose and light. Your heart is beating evenly, your lungs gently expanding and contracting. Your body's systems are fluid, languid, all is well. You are in a safe place, your surroundings protecting you, freeing you to transcend your physical place and go to a place of the mind, to take a journey of the mind.

Your mind and your body are easy to attune, one integrated with the other. But it is your mind which is the stronger, and your mind is the key to the realm we are about to enter. You are receptive to my words, to the images I will suggest. You can summon memories of smells and tastes from the past. You can see faces from the past, faces of the future. You are at one with body and mind, and you are at one with space and time. Feel yourself lift up out of your own body, to rise out of the room you're in a go up into the sky. Look around at the clouds, the clear blue stretching out and up in every direction.

Lower yourself down now, in complete control of your mind-self as your descend. You are lighter than air as you return to your room, your body, entering as if sitting down into a comfortable old chair. You lean back, body perfectly comfortable, serenity and tranquility flooding through you. You are open and ready, your mind is eager, my voice is your guide.

For a long time, you have been acting and feeling in ways that are not your own, ways that have taken you away from your own, natural self. You have relied more and more on eating to help you through the negative feelings which you have been experiencing, and have done so to such an extent that you deny yourself your own true feelings.

Nobody feels on top of the world all the time. There will be days that could be better for you. It is only by experiencing some of life's lows that you can enjoy and appreciate life's highs. Blotting out your feelings with overeating does not solve anything, it only makes things worse. That is why you have decided that you have had enough of overeating, and you want help with that old problems of yours.

Focus on a part of your life that you feel happy with. Enjoy remembering some of the good things that happened to you, something that made you feel confident. Reflect on an achievement, or on some praise you received. Note how you feel; confident, proud happy. and allow those good feelings to grow stronger, while you relax, and let go.

And when those good feelings come, take a very deep breath, hold it, and squeeze your hand into a fist. Your subconscious mind memorizes these good feelings. You are imprinting this feeling, this moment, into your memory, into your body's memory, into your muscle memory. It is as if you have driven that feeling into your hand, an invisible diamond in your palm. Let it be the storage place for that memory, for that feeling. When you wish to enjoy this feeling again, all you have to do is take a long deep breath and squeeze your hand into a fist. You will release that feeling from the diamond in your palm and your mind will access that memory.

Envision yourself in a situation where you would reach for your first sugary snack. Note where you are, what you are doing, who is with you, if anyone is there, use your imagination to remember it with as much detail as you can manage.

Note your feelings as you reach for the fridge. Think of the feeling of helplessness you have always had, and how those feelings have affected your life. Now envision yourself walking away and looking out the window. Take a deep breath in through your nose and squeeze the other hand into a tight fist while you remember those good, confident positive feelings. Savor their familiarity, how they make you feel that you can meet any challenge, that you are the very best and strongest you that there is.

You feel good. It is good to be confident, and to know that you are finally free from your old, addictive way of life. You are free of the burden of having to eat constantly. You are free to move ahead with your life, to experience the highs and the lows. Knowing this will help you appreciate it when things get better.

Envision an alternative activity. It does not matter what it is just as long as it is a break from the norm. What are you imagining? Skydiving? Swimming in a turquoise sea? Do you see your slim body, tawny and muscular, as you glide through the water?

You are changing. Your old ways of behaving and thinking are improving, you are in command, you are taking charge, you are in control. You are free as a bird, you are free from the addictive way of life, and yes, there will be moments when you feel pain, but these moments will get less, and you will appreciate the pleasurable things in life, the little things that make you smile and feel good.

You can glide like a dolphin through an azure sea. You can fly up out of your own body and hover with the clouds. Your mind and your body work together, to take you anywhere and to face anything, to do anything. You are open and receptive, your mind able to conjure anything and any place. You can feel it, smell it, sense it.

Envision that you are standing at the bottom of a small flight of stairs, leading up into an attic. There are ten steps leading gently up and you feel drawn towards climbing the stairs to explore the contents of this attic. With each step, climb toward the attic, become more deeply and comfortably relaxed.

Take the first step and feel yourself becoming even more deeply relaxed.

Two … three … ascending higher … four … you feel light, floaty, and you are more deeply relaxed than before.

Five … you reach a small landing and turn as the stairs take you in another direction.

Six … note a pleasant familiar aroma of wood. It is almost like being at a carpenter's workshop. Seven … you are surprised by the warmth as you ascend.

Eight … nine … and ten.

You are at the top of the stairs and you note a door in front of you. The door is locked, and there are two keys hanging by the side of the door. Take one of the keys and slip it into the lock of the attic door.

It fits and you unlock the attic door, opening it carefully and turning on the light. Note are beautiful dark oak beams running across the ceiling of the attic, and when you look down you see rickety old floorboards that creak ever so slightly beneath your feet.

Just to your left is a large old brown, trunk (like a treasure chest). It is bound by leather straps, fastened by buckles.

You are curious about what the trunk contains. Undo the straps. The trunk is padlocked. You try the spare key you took from the side of the door. The trunk unlocks and you lift the lid and take a peek inside.

It is crammed with memorabilia; positive memories from times gone by, your hopes and dreams for the future, valuable lessons that you learned as a youngster, inspirational thoughts and ideas and dreams, and images of your ideal self, the person you will be when you have achieved your goal of a slimmer and healthier body.

You rummage through the trunk, musing over your childhood dreams. You admire the concept of a slimmer you; the you who is able to enjoy the activities that you love and live the life that you desire.

I will be quiet for a moment as you look through these memories and dreams.

There are so many memories here, from times that you thought were completely forgotten; so many good and happy experiences and so much joy for a future that is yet to arrive.

Your subconscious mind realizes that you can achieve your true potential, having succeeded already in so many things.

Select a memory that is associated with positive, happy and confident feelings, perhaps a time when you were your ideal weight and shape or maybe some other time when you had achieved a goal that made you feel good.

I'll be quite for a moment as you re-experience that situation in every detail.

Note how you looked at that time; your hairstyle, your clothes, the surrounding environment. Note who you are with (if anyone) and what you are doing. Remember any remarks that you or anyone else may have made (a compliments perhaps) that increase these good feelings.

There may even be a certain aroma or something else that you associate with this memory. I do not know what this memory is, but what I do know is that it is very special to you.

Enjoy the confident and positive feelings while I am quiet for a moment. Before we move on, label your experience, like the title of a movie or a book. It is time to descend the stairs from the attic of the past. Would be lovely to bring some of those positive experiences back?

You could place them into that bag lying near the door of the attic. Or you could put them in a jar. Or you could just keep them in a deep corner of your mind, or somewhere close to your heart.

Once you have saved those happy memories, close the lid of the trunk. Lock it and buckle the straps. Bring your container holding those confident memories to bring back with you. Close and lock the door to the attic and descend the stairs, counting as we go down.

Ten ... coming slowly down. Nine ... you are leaving the aroma of the wood behind you. Eight ...

you are bringing those experiences back, you have them with you always. Seven ... you are feeling even more relaxed, more comfortable, more confident. Six ... five ... you pause for a second or two on the landing before continuing down the stairway.

Four ... three ... two ... one ... you are leaving the attic behind. You know that you can return on your own when you want, whenever you wish; to rediscover other valuable experiences that can help you in the present and in the future.

You know what it is to be healthy and slim. You have happy dreams and memories of your ideal self. You can achieve your goal with the power of your subconscious mind.

You find it easy to say *no* to anything standing in the way of achieving your goal weight. In the past, certain drinks or foods were considered temptations. But you feel and respond in a different way now. Everything is different now and it will go on being different in the future.

Something inside you has changed. You have all the motivation and determination you need to succeed, and you do succeed. You have succeeded at a good many things in the past. You will succeed again. If you need to, you may remind yourself of your many achievements just by recalling the label of your happiest memory from your chest in the memory attic.

Relax. Enjoy your memory in detail, with all the sounds, colors, smells. Focus on the good feelings and thoughts. Focus on the feelings of accomplishment, achievement, the pride of attaining your goals. Savor the positive sensations related to that good and happy time of your life.

It will be exciting for you to see how rapidly these good feelings return to you; boosting your confidence, increasing your determination and motivation to succeed and to achieve your ideal weight and shape. It will be gratifying to be able to wear stylish clothes of a smaller size. You will enjoy feeling comfortable in your own skin and being content and happy and with your life and with yourself.

Whenever you want or need to, just recall your key word, the label you gave to your happy time. This lets you be confident and to feel good about yourself. You are now more motivated and determined to succeed.

It will be especially exciting when, in five or six months, you look back on your trip to the attic. You will be sure that you are well on your way. You may even have achieved your goal already, having reached your desired weight and shape.

You will realize that you were always able to be the person you wanted to be; your healthier, slimmer self. You will be able to use your own life experiences and realize your dreams. You can make these dreams come true in the way you wanted them to come true, and you'll do it by using the power of your subconscious mind.

This makes it easy to maintain your true size and shape. You already have the key to success (your key word). Think that word in your mind and you will reinforce these good feelings.

You find that something you may have thought was impossible has become as simple as one-two-three. You also note that, from this moment forward, new opportunities open up to you. Your mind is open, receptive to changes at a much deeper level. These are changes which can benefit you in countless ways.

You can become a great achievers; because whatever your mind can conceive, you can achieve. Reaching your true, ideal shape and weight is just the start of a life-changing adventure.

With every breath you take and every word that I say, any and all stresses, tensions, worries or doubts about your ability to lose weight are disappearing. You are free of them now, weightless. There is nothing to constrain you, nothing weighing you down. You feel stronger than ever, more attuned to the connection of body and mind. You are secure, confident, certain that you can face even the most intimidating challenges with ease and aplomb. Remember that your friends and family know this too, they look to you for a better example, to help them be better people. You may think that they judge you, and if they do they do it with mercy and positivity. They judge you to be a good and worthy person, imperfect as all people are. And that support inspires you to show them just how close to perfection a person may get. You know you probably won't actually ever achieve perfection, but striving for it will get you closer than anything else will. You know that, and you know how much effort will be called upon. And you know you can muster that effort, that strength and power, that and so much more.

You have made a decision to take the journey to your ideal shape and weight. It is easy for you to stay on the path, doing all the things you must do to achieve your goal.

You eat smaller, healthier portions of food. You leave food on your plate without realizing it, without even thinking about it.

If you have ever snacked between meals then you already know you do not want or need to snack anymore. You have uncovered the secrets of snacking, the disguised motivators which you never knew before. But you know them now. Now you are better-equipped to change your behavior. Because you know why it has to be changed, and you know that you are the only one who can change it. You enjoy changing it. You enjoy the feeling of control, the rewards of self-discipline. You are the champion of your own body, and you relish being called upon to do your duty. You are looking after your body by exercising when you can. You are providing it is safe and appropriate for you to do so.

And your subconscious mind is helping you do this, helping you around the clock. You trust in your powerful subconscious mind. You know that it will not let you down.

It is time for you to return to normal, conscious awareness. You will be eager and ready to begin the journey toward achieving a healthier, slimmer body and a stronger, more powerful mind.

Remember that, as you go about your daily life, your mind-life also goes on. Your mind-self and your life-self must be partners, working in unity for the greater good of your general wellness. These suggestions, and others in other sessions, should remain with you. Let them linger. Live your life the way you would in your mind-realm; with a sense of control, of strength.

These suggestions are firmly embedded in your subconscious mind and grow stronger every day. They grow stronger by the day, stronger by the hour, stronger by the minute. You find that every time you listen to my voice. It gets easier to relax and to enter hypnosis. The suggestions will have more benefit. They are now a permanent part of your new reality.

Remember your key word, the label that you gave to your happy memory. Repeat it to yourself if and when you encounter a situation that might have prevented you from reaching your goal in the past.

Your key word is the key to the trunk, the treasure chest in the attic containing all your happiest experiences and memories. You can unlock it whenever you like to recover those feelings with the power of your subconscious mind.

But you can also leave it behind, move ahead without feeling weighed down by anything from the past, good or bad. You may use these things, draw strength from them. But true strength is in what you do today, not what happened before. You will always be able to handle any challenges from this point onward, no matter where you go or what you do. You will go on strengthening your powers until nothing dare stand in your way.

If you need the past, it is there for you. If you need the future, it is waiting. The present is where the two meet, and that is only now. Even the present cannot contain you. The present is ever-changing, just as you are ever-changing. You are all things, past, present, and future. Connect them as you did your body and your mind, let them work together. Let the past guide the present and help create the future instead of burdening the present and destroying the future. You are the champion of your body and of your life, of your future. You must create it, protect it, nurture it the way you do your body and your mind. Do not let others sully it, do not let yourself sully it either. You are stronger than that, you are stronger than yourself.

In a moment, I'm going to count to five. At the count of five, you will be awake. Beautiful feelings will flow through you, confident and calm thoughts filling your mind.

These confident and calm thoughts and feelings will stay with you. They remain within you, becoming stronger as the days goes by.

One … two … you're coming back slowly. Three … take a comforting and comfortable breath. Four … your eyelids are fluttering now. Five … your eyes open, you are wide awake, mind and body returning to normal conscious awareness.

Now let's relax and reflect. How did it feel going down those stairs? Are you comfortable with your key word? Do you feel ready and empowered to lose the weight? You should see now that you have incredible powers, powers of the mind, which you may never have realized were in you before. Now you know what kind of strength you can access. You can walk through any door, descend even the darkest staircase without fear. The demons which have plagued you have no power over you now. And if they do, or seem to, that power will soon recede as your own power advances. Everything about your life may well have changed, even if you do not realize it.

That is good. There's much you are only coming to realize, only now beginning to discover; about yourself, your body, your life. Keep learning, keep growing, keep trying.

Emotional Eating

Close your eyes and envision lying in a hot bubble bath. Feel the warm water caressing you, easing your tensions and relaxing your body, soothing you all over. You feel comfortable, your limbs and body are heavy. You are savoring the luxury of having nothing to do, nothing but to relaxing and just letting go.

Sense the warmth and that heaviness spreading over your entire body from your toes and your feet slowly up into the legs. Feel that warmth as it flows into your belly, abdomen rising and falling. Your breathing is regular and calm as your chest relaxes and your shoulders become limp and loose and relaxed.

Relax your arms as the comfort and warmth flow down from your shoulders. Savor the feeling, enjoy it.

Your throat and neck also relax, so do your little facial muscles. Your eyes become heavy, almost closed. But you can still focus on a single bubble in that bath, one particular bubble in all the thousands, the one that reflects beautiful colors from the sunlight which streams in through the window.

That little bubble contains every color in the rainbow, deep and pristine and clear. The reds are bursting, the blue deep and rich, the yellow hot and the green soothing.

Envision that bubble growing, expanding, more delicate than it was before. Note that the heaviness is gone and you can envision leaving your body through the crown of your head and floating up over the tub.

Float down and toward the bubble, head first and as your head reaches the bubble. The bubble turns inside out and engulfs you, your entire body. Now you are surrounded by gossamer film of color. You are floating back up and into a clear blue sky. You're lifting higher, not doing or feeling or thinking, only being.

You go higher, and you feel more relaxed and more comfortable. You are protected and safe in your bubble.

I will be silent so you can absorb the beauty and peace of this heightened awareness. When you do hear my voice once more, it will seem to be coming from outside the bubble. Your subconscious mind will be open, receptive to what you hear.

As you drift down deeper into hypnosis, your mind becomes receptive and open and to everything I say and everything I suggest. Your subconscious mind will listen intently. It will absorb any suggestions that are beneficial of your overall wellbeing and good health.

These suggestions will go deep. They will make a lasting impression. They will be ingrained in your mind, indelible. As these suggestions sink into your unconscious mind, they become a part of your life. They will influence the way you feel, the way you think, even the way you eat.

For a long while, you have been using food to cope with negative feelings. Whether these feelings are the result of sadness, loneliness, boredom, depression, anxiousness, frustration or anger, it does not matter.

When you eat when you are not hungry, you know it will take much longer to lose those extra pounds. If you look to food for comfort, that comfort will be short-lived. It solves no long-term problems, not for you or for anyone.

Deep down, you are aware of this. If food actually provided a true source of comfort, you would feel great all the time.

Emotional eating worsens your issues by generating extra weight that you do not want or need. You are learning that eating when you are emotional is only a temporary distraction. You start looking for healthier distracts.

You have full and complete control of the united efforts of body and mind, working together toward your overall wellness. You know they can meet any challenge, even the united efforts of emotional frustration and the temptation to overeat. They are also working together, to keep you on a downward spiral of mental and psychological decline. Your weight will go up while your confidence goes down. But your allied efforts are stronger. You will not be tempted or beguiled by these interlopers into your life. What are the reasons for your emotional tumult? How should you best deal with them?

You may begin by writing down your thoughts and feelings in a diary or journal. You realize this will help you to get them out of your head. You may recognize and identify the triggers which used to make you seek comfort from food.

You might call a relative or close friend for support. By sharing your problems, you find that they seem far less significant. Talking on the phone is also a welcome distraction from food. And it isn't polite to eat and talk at the same time, so you forgo that trip to the cupboard.

Clear your fridge and cupboards of junk food like cakes and chocolates. You substitute them for healthy snacks like fresh vegetables and fruit and low-fat food. You are done with emotional eating and you explore other activities which give you that good feeling.

You have many choices in life. You may join a club and meet other people. You may watch a feel-good movie. You might spend extra time cleaning your home, realizing that the exercise will help you lose weight while the smell of cleaning products will stifle your appetite.

You accept yourself as the unique person you are. You love your body. You like what goes into it.

You treat it well by eating only small amounts of healthy food and exercising as much as you can. You treat yourself with respect and you expect others to treat you with respect in the same way. You have earned it and you deserve it.

Your emotions may wear the face of someone else, somebody who hurt you in the past. Picture that person's face, envision it. Perhaps your own face is the one you see, your disappointments turning against your own bad judgments and past mistakes. Either way, you are stronger now, strong enough to forgive. Forgive that other person. Even more difficult, forgive yourself. Forgive yourself for whatever you may have done and for whatever you may be feeling.

You also accept that your emotions are an essential part of your whole personality and you find constructive ways of expressing yourself. They are the voice of what is best about you; sensitivity, empathy, humanity. Your emotions are insights into your higher self. Accept them, embrace them, but do not let them control you. You do not let your emotions control you. Like your body, which you love and accept, you likewise love and accept your emotions. But you have gained control over your body so your body and mind can work together and not be at odds. So too must your mind and your emotions work together, and it must the subconscious and the conscious mind which makes that happen. It is your mind which makes that happen.

You exercise more, slowly at first if necessary. Your brain releases those feel-good hormones to make you feel calm, happy, more able to cope with the various challenges and issues that might crop up. You get stronger every day, in mind and body, strong enough to handle your emotions as you never could before. You do not need food to help you cope with feelings other than genuine hunger. The next time you feel emotional, when you might reach for the cupboard out of habit, you stop and reflect on the things I have been saying today.

You are not hungry, so there is no need for you to eat. Before you were eating just to have something to do, or to work out your emotions. There are plenty of other things to do with your time. There are other ways to work out your emotions. You put everything into creating a happier, richer, more fulfilling life. You can do everything you ever wanted to do plus so much more.

You no longer link emotions with eating. You eat merely when you are hungry. Your life is becoming so much more fulfilling now that you have no need to eat just for the sake of it.

You are not eating when you are emotional. You find that you have more energy, more vitality. You exercise more. You enjoy using your body. And the more you use it, the healthier your body becomes.

You need less food. You want less food. You have no taste for the junk food you used to eat. You have no interest in fatty, greasy foods that will damage your alley, your body. You have distaste for the sugary, processed foods you used to rely on. Your body craves better foods, nutritional foods. You mind knows your brain needs the too, and you are happy to do what you can for your body, your mind, your best self.

Because not only do you deserve it, but you demand it. You've become too strong to be manipulated by things like memories or emotions. The unity of your body and mind is too strong a bond to be violated. It is too strong an alliance to be thwarted.

Look at yourself in the mirror and you'll see for yourself. Look at your body, leaner for having lost all those excess pounds. You are firmer, slimmer, toned. You are glowing with vitality and health. Note what you are wearing and how everything looks so good on your trim body.

Look at your face, with a brighter glow from the healthier foods, the better nights' sleep, the calm and repose from the yoga and meditation, the shine of inner peace. This is the real you, slowly rising from the ashes of the old you. This is the best you, the person you were meant to be. Little by little, the true self emerges from the illusions and frustrations of the old.

Your mind and body meet with your own approval. You are gratified and glad that you cut the link between eating and all those negative, emotional thoughts. You are proud to be a person who is strong enough to do such impressive things. You are accumulating accomplishments every day; with every pound lost, with every good night's rest, with every day's fasting. You have learned what you need and you are taking step to get them. That is something most others can never accomplish. You will never allow anybody to distort your opinion of yourself again. You are great and you are only getting better, every day and in every way.

You have an image of your ideal life, your ideal self, your ideal future. You have envisioned them, they are waiting for you. You know the effort it will take to cross the Rubicon and get to the other side, where paradise awaits; your personal paradise. And you know now that nobody can stop you, nothing can obstruct you. Nothing can or will weigh you down, not any more. It may have happened in the past, but things have changed. You have changed. And nothing will ever be the way it was before.

Every day you are moving closer to this new image. Every day you are more determined and you are more motivated to achieve your goal. Instead of eating in an attempt to fill some emotional void, you find more constructive ways of dealing with your feelings. You soon see a slimmer, happier you.

These suggestions are embedded in your subconscious mind. They grow stronger day by day. They are deeply embedded in your subconscious mind, where they will take effect at the earliest opportunity.

In a moment, I'm going to count from one to five and at the count of five, you'll be wide awake. One … two … three, returning to consciousness now. Four … your eyes are fluttering, opening. And … five.

Now let's relax and reflect. Has your hunger subsided? Do you feel strong enough to fight the pangs of hunger when they arrive? Do you fee properly empowered? Have you discovered a new relationship to food? Do you have a greater understanding of your strength? Do you have a better comprehension of your own emotional distress, and how you may be misguiding your own emotional expression? Food has real value, life-saving value. But it is not meant to be abused. It has no powers over the mind other than to befuddle and confuse. It is crucial to maintain control of the mind over the body, and this means control of reason over emotion. We said earlier that reason is a function of the mind, but emotion more a function of the body. So now you are well-poised to take greater control of your emotions by asserting the power of reason. You are better prepared to deal with your emotions in a constructive way, not a destructive way. Now you can face them head-on and re-establish a healthier relationship with your food ... and yourself.

Self-Image

Close your eyes and take a deep breath. Feel your body and mind strengthen their bond with one another, creating your best mind-self. You are confident that you know what you are doing here. There is nothing dubious, nothing odd, nothing surprising now about these journeys into the world of the mind and beyond, all the way to the stars if you so choose. You are experienced, you are strong. You have come a long way in your journey and learned much. Your instincts are sharper, your insight is deeper. The eyes of your heart can see what the eyes of your head have turned from for so many years.

But even time is your domain, to use at your will. You are a traveler in time, into your own past and your own future. You are your body's champion. You are a conqueror. And now you lean back and relax, preparing to set forth again. Let my words guide you further down our life path, into the realm of the self. You travel inward even as you transcend. You will leave your body even as you have gotten closer to it.

You have been forging a new relationship with your body, becoming its alley. It needs you to function at its best, to make the best decisions for feeding it or not, what and when. You now have the strength to make better choices, your mind well-able to take control, to lead where your body will readily follow.

You are ready to be kinder to yourself, to see yourself in a new and flattering light, a forgiving light. You are receptive, ready to take on any challenge, even the challenge of your own body. But you have done this before, and you know that you are more than able to prevail; for mind, body, and soul.

Take a deep breath and hold it, then release it in a cleansing exhalation. Breathe in and hold it, let it out again. Savor the relaxed feeling, the sense of ease that fills you. Nothing can stand in your way and nothing can hold you back.

Picture yourself outside in your favorite place in nature. It might be a tropical beach, it might be a lovely garden, or perhaps you could picture yourself laying back on a boat sailing on a beautiful river. It does not matter where you are, as long as it feels good to you.

Nod your head when you are thinking of that special place.

It is a beautiful day. The sky is a beautiful blue, very clear. It is a warm summer's day. A dazzling sun hangs in the sky. It is so bright and colorful that you want to close your eyes and feel the warmth of the sun on your body. Envision this.

You can direct the sun around your body. As you realize this, you direct the light from the sun over your face. You can feel the warmth of the light from the sun on your face, just relaxing those muscles around the eyes and the nose and the mouth.

Your facial muscles flatten as they relax, and you let go. It is a beautiful day. You move the light from the sun into your throat area, feeling the warmth of the light from the sun in your throat, relaxing all those muscles, letting go. And the sunlight moves into the shoulders and across the shoulders, making them feel loose and limp and comfortable.

You feel relaxed, comfortable and at peace with the world. Direct the light from the sun down the right arm, from the shoulders to the tips of the fingers, the right arm begins to relax and let go, relax and let go. It is a beautiful feeling to be here right. The warmth of the light from the sun penetrates nerves and bones and muscles of that right arm.

It is a beautiful day. Move the sun over to the left arm and guide the light from the sun down and up the left arm, from the top of the shoulders to your fingertips. Your left arm is relaxing, becoming heavy, and you feel even more comfortable and relaxed. Move the light across and into your chest area and relax the chest and all the muscles there. Relax your stomach, let that relaxation spread to your hips and your thighs and over to your right leg.

Relax your right leg. Let it feel comfortable and relaxed. Move the light from the sun down the right leg, up and down, from the top of the hips to the tips of the toes, and the right leg relaxes, and let go.

It is a beautiful day. Move the light into your left leg. Move it up and down your left leg, from the top of your hips to the tips of your toes. Your left leg relaxes, releases tension, it lets go. Your whole body is totally relaxed, from the top of your head to the tips of your toes.

As your body relaxes, so does your mind. As your mind relaxes, note that the sun is going down. The sun is going down, slowly descending. The sky is alight with colors, crimson and purple with yellow and blue streaks. It is a beautiful evening. Your mind lets go, releases all the stress of the day. You … just … let … go.

The sun goes further down, over the horizon, until the sky is black, like black velvet. And twinkling up there in the sky is a single twinkling star. Keep your mind focused on that star. Nothing else matters but this beautiful single, bright star in the sky.

It is a beautiful night. You feel safe, comfortable, relaxed. You feel at peace with the

Universe. Envision yourself moving toward that star in the sky, moving up, and up and up.

Your body is weightless as you lift to the star, ascending to greater heights. As the star grows, you realize you are getting close to it … closer … closer. It gets bigger … brighter.

Then, all at once, you *are* that star in the night sky. That is right. *You* are that silver solitary star in the night sky. You become the star and the star is you. You are one, back from where you came. And it is a beautiful star. You are a beautiful star.

Let your mind go, set it free to wander. As you drift into this restful, calm feeling, I am going to talk about your self-image, which is somewhat different, slightly distorted from the way other people see you. I know you have difficulty in accepting other people's opinions of how you look when they tell you that you really do look good.

You see yourself as being fat and unattractive. No matter how many times you are told otherwise, you find it hard (if not impossible_ to believe. So you wind up walking through life with your eyes closed to the opportunities around you, oblivious to the rewards which could be yours for the taking.

But the world sees a better you. The world sees the attractive you which even you deny. The world sees the lean, attractive you, or the hearty, playful you. The world sees the person it wants to get to know. The world has never seen the person that you imagine yourself to be. That person does not exist, only in your mind. But your mind is now stronger, and combined with the strength in your body, you cannot be stopped. With your mind and body united, working together, you can see what the rest of the world sees. That's the real you, the better you. The person you imagine does not exist, but the person the world sees does exist. That's you. And you, mind and body strong, are no match for some imagined shadow of your true self, a distorted, funhouse-mirror reflection of reality.

You are missing out on so much. You may find it hard to accept compliments. You may shy away from some places or activities because you are afraid that you do not you look as good as other people there will.

Being attractive or slim is not necessarily an advantage. But not believing in yourself can certainly prove a handicap; if you do not believe in yourself, how will others be able to believe in you? Let us improve your self-image, to help you to see yourself as you truly are. You are going to learn how to accept that you already are an attractive, sensitive, intelligent person with a well-proportioned body and a self-assured, confident style.

You do not have to be ashamed of your body. You can and should be proud of your body, to accept yourself for the person you are.

I know you tend to compare yourself unfavorably to others. It can seem hard to accept your own body when all you see in the media are super-slim models and celebrities. You might think that this is the normal way to look. You have strived all of your life to attain similar physiques by dieting or extreme workouts.

But you do not see or feel how starved and image-obsessed celebrities often become.

Everything in their lives seems to revolve around their own self-image and how others perceive them and if they fail to live up to their self-imposed expectations this can often lead to disastrous consequences. They may feel under constant pressure to maintain unreasonable expectations and this can impact upon their personal life as they feel their privacy has been invaded. It is an ongoing cycle. Stress invariably begins to build up.

Others may be influenced by their images because they are bombarded with perfection with every magazine or popular film and that is all they tend to see. But the reality is that those celebrities often yearn for ordinary, normal lives like most of us enjoy.

You can set your own realistic standards without having to conform to other people's lofty expectations. You can concentrate on truly worthwhile achievements and becoming a contributing member of society. You can become a person who gives something back rather than who constantly seeks to bask in artificial adulation.

Focus on your positive qualities; things about you or your achievements that you are proud of, qualities which endear you to the people who matter most in your life. Focus on your eyes, the windows of your soul. Focus on your smile. Every smile is lovely, all eyes are truth and truth is beauty. Think about the new leanness of your torso after your fasting, diet, and exercise. Think about your new flexibility from the yoga practices you've been doing. Enjoy the new looseness you feel, the looks you've been getting from others. Do not be blind to them, do not turn away from happy happenstance. You deserve it and it will come to you. Do not ignore or deny it. Embrace it, embrace your eyes and your smile and your ever-improving body and mind. Embrace everything you have to offer, everything that you are.

Allow these to fill your mind as I'm quiet for a moment, and when you hear my voice again, your subconscious mind will be open and ready to embark on a short journey with me.

Now let's go for a walk along a path that represents your life. You will recognize some of the achievements you have accomplished. These could be described as quite small, such as learning to ride a bike, reading a book, and so forth. Others may be more important achievements, such as learning a language or getting a new job. It does not matter how small or large those achievements were, they are all there on your path of life.

When you are ready, we will begin at the very beginning of your beginning; your conception. The moment of conception, which has been caught on camera, is an explosion of sparks of light, like a tiny, natural fireworks display.

Even as a fetus, you achieved milestones as you reached crucial developmental stages until you were ready for birth. You are already on your own path of life where you continue to develop. As a baby, you mastered important skills like sitting up, crawling, feeding yourself, communicating. As a small child you had much to learn, yet you learned those new skills. See yourself, see that you have grown up and started at school. You made friends, you learned how to socialize; perhaps you met your first best friend or another person you played with at this time.

Walk along your path of life and note all which you have achieved. Acknowledge your attainments and successes, appreciate what a human being you already are. As you make your journey, note mirrors that reflect back all the positive contributions you have made throughout your life.

Catch a glimpse of yourself in the mirror. You may think: "Yes, that is me. That is what I did and I am proud of that accomplishment." You know and appreciate how there are many more important things than appearance, such as personality, kindness, respectfulness toward others.

You are also quite happy with the way that you look. You tell yourself, "I am great. I genuinely like myself. I love myself. I accept myself totally and unreservedly for the unique person I am." As you continue on the path you will see that there are some turning points on your path; major life changes.

See yourself walking this path, happy and calm. Note a bonfire a little bit. Tell me when you reach the bonfire.

You have travelled far and you still have a long way to go.

Give a little consideration to any negative comments or thoughts you have experienced or which you may have received about the way that you look. They may only have been words, and even though they lacked substance they were enough to make you emotionally upset.

It is time to reject those thoughts, feelings, emotions, and comments. Take each for what it is. Study it for a second or two to reassure yourself that it is not relevant to you and then toss it onto the bonfire. If anyone has ever put you down in any way, insulted you, or teasingly said something to upset you, examine those comments briefly before throwing them into the fire.

See your old hurts, sadness, insecurities, humiliation, anger, or embarrassment. Look at each one carefully before tossing them onto the bonfire and watch while they burn.

Remind yourself, "I am fine. I like myself. I love myself. I accept myself entirely for the unique person that I am." If there is anything else preventing you from loving and accepting yourself as the person you are, then get rid of it. It does not have any place in your life. All those harmful and negative emotions and feelings are gone. You truly and completely accept yourself for the unique individual that you are.

Acceptance does not mean you become complacent. You still strive to accomplish goals and satisfy desires, just like anybody does. But you are able to prioritize what is important to you and what is not.

As the negativities have all gone up in smoke, you note another mirror. Step over to the mirror and examine yourself from head to toe. See yourself standing tall, shoulders back, head held high and a confident smile on your face. And tell yourself, "I love myself, and I respect myself. I have a good body. I have a healthy body. I love my body. I accept my body. From now on, I recognize what is important to me and that is what matters.

Other people's opinions are just that; their opinions. If they are offensive or insulting, I can find it strangely amusing as it means that deep down, they are the insecure ones with problems about their body.

You accept these suggestions because you know they make sense. You know they are the truth, and truth is beauty. You love and respect your body. From now on you trust yourself. You trust your intuition, you trust your subconscious mind. You know that you are a good and worthwhile person who has achieved a lot in life. You are person who is admired by those around you. You are an example of personal excellence to others. You are secret desire of people and you do not even know it. You will likely never know it. But that is okay. Your confidence and best self will find what you need, who you need. You will no longer be distracted by what you imagine others may think of you either way. You are following your own path. You have your eye on a shining star over velvet-black sky. You reach for that star, you reach that star, you are that start. You will continue on your path without concern for what others think or say about you.

We will talk more about it, I will make suggestions and these suggestions will be firmly embedded in your subconscious mind. They will grow stronger every day. They will become a part of your psyche, a part of your psychology. And in so being, they become a part of your mind-self and a part of your best self, body and mind. You will be open to the suggestions, mind and body both relaxed and alert. You are at the apex of your mind's powers and your body's strength.

In a moment, I will count the numbers from one to five and at the count of five, you will be fully refreshed and alert. You will be ready to allow these suggestions to work in your life. One … two … three, you're coming slowly back. Four … your eyelids are fluttering. Five ... your eyes are open, you are wide awake, your mind and body are returning to normal.

Now let's relax and reflect. Do you feel better about your body? Do you feel more confident? Do you have more compassion for yourself, a greater appreciation of your own beauty, inward and outward? Do you feel that you can access that appreciation with greater ease? Have you gained a greater understanding of what people go through and suffer through in order to embrace that false sense of glamor and superiority?

All things in nature are beautiful. Beauty truly is in the eye of the beholder. Now your own eyes are open wider than they were, keener to observe the hidden beauty in all things, especially yourself. Hold onto that new perspective, using any of the techniques in the book to do so. Make it your mantra during meditation, envision it when you fast or diet. This is the idealized you that you're working toward, the better life and perfect future which is your goal, and to which you are more than entitled.

Keep working, it is getting closer every day, in every way, and you're getting better and better.

Interrupted Sleep Relaxation

Ease your body and mind and relax. Leave your troubles behind you. You feel more at ease. It is okay if your mind wanders to pleasant but distracting thought. Your inner mind continues to listen. It enjoys the sense of harmony, peace, and tranquility that grows and develops inside you.

You know those feelings that you have when sleeping soundly, how you sometimes wish that you could just be left to sleep. Remember how you felt laying on a lawn or on a beach in the sun. You recall drifting in and out of sleep, yawning, and wanting nothing more than to stay just where you were.

Remember the comforting feeling of being a child, snug in your bed. You were safe, you were secure, you were looked after. Your childhood challenges may have seemed like a lot, but you can see them now for the mere trifles that they were. You were warm and comfortable and taken care of, a refuge that adult life rarely offers. You had no real responsibilities, as you do now. You faced no real risks, as you do now. Your life was simple, uncomplicated. Recall those warm, comforting feelings, of your mother's loving embrace and of a warm dinner in your belly. Sleep was a refuge then as it is today, necessary for body, mind, and soul. Sleep refreshes the mind as it give the body a chance to fast and to renew. Every morning you wake up, you are born anew.

Think about those rainy nights when you were a child, snuggled up warm. Reflect on those summer days when you could blissfully sleep in. Use your powerful subconscious mind to conjure the smells, the sights, your childhood bedroom. What was hanging on the walls? Were there pets in the room? Can you smell the cedar shavings of the hamster cage, or the briny scent of the fish food?

Relax and let your senses come alive. Be open and receptive, your mind ready to take you where you need and want to be. There's nothing stopping you, nothing threatening you. You are free. You are strong. You are in total control. You are in control of your body and mind. You are in control of your world, of all worlds.

You *are* all worlds.

You are free. You are free to travel where you wish, whenever you wish. You can travel to wherever you wish, to envision your ideal self in your ideal future. You can go to the past and forgive and let go, then release it forever. You can clean out the cupboards of your emotions, you can tell what is truth and what is a lie, an illusion meant to beguile. You cannot be fooled. You cannot be beguiled. You cannot be controlled. You cannot be contained. You cannot be constrained. You will not be controlled. You will not be contained. You will not be constrained.

I'm going to count slowly back from ten to zero and as I do, you find that you relax more and more with every number. You feel just now just as deeply relaxed as you did then.

Ten ... feel yourself descending. Nine ... you're drifting lazily. Eight ... you're relaxing even more. Seven ... you're going deeper. Six ... deeper still. Five ... you're halfway to total body relaxation. Four ... that comfortable feeling is returning to your arms, legs, torso. Three, two ... you're almost there. One ... zero.

Now you're looking up into a gorgeous night sky and that you can see a star in the distance. You can see one beautiful, solitary, silver star, shining down out of a velvety black night sky. That star is countless millions of miles away. You focus on that one solitary star. Note how it sparkles. You're even more relaxed now, more peaceful, calmer.

Envision yourself rising out of your body, drawn to that star. You move toward that star, through space and time and through the earth's stratosphere, passing planets and comets, passing through other galaxies, as you get closer to the star.

The nearer you get, the larger and brighter it is and the more comfortable and relaxed you are. Finally, you arrive at the star, it is right there in front of you ... one solitary silver star. Now you are on the star, *in* the star ... and the star is in you.

Now you *are* the star, the star is *you.*

Go deeper into a gentle hypnotic rest. Note the beautiful stairway in your star, with hundreds of sterling steps descending. You walk down the stairs, very nearly floating, your feet not touching the stairs at all. The word *relax* is written on each step. As you descend. you become even more comfortable, more at ease and relaxed. and at ease.

You're becoming sleepier, drifting deeper. From time to time, you may feel as if you are drifting off to sleep because you are so relaxed ... so ... relaxed.

For a while now, you know that you have been having trouble going back to sleep once you have been awakened and I know that you need to be fully alert once you awaken in order to deal with the situation in hand.

However, once you have dealt with the situation you have probably found that the harder you try to go back to sleep, the harder it is. This is known as *the law of reversed effect*. We are going to reverse that situation again by using a different technique.

Instead of trying to get back to sleep, you are going to learn how to put yourself into a hypnotic trance. And who knows? This may lead to sleep. But if it does not, you will still receive the same benefit as being asleep; because one hour of hypnosis is worth eight hours of quality sleep.

When your sleep is interrupted and it is time for you to go back to your bed, make yourself as comfortable as possible. Begin by imagining that you asked to perform a particularly unpleasant task. This chore is something you do not want to do, something you would go way out of your way to avoid doing, if possible.

If you were asleep, you would not need to respond to the request. So pretend that you are asleep. Match the breathing pattern that you adapt when you are just falling asleep; slowly, rhythmically, deeply, evenly, breathing in slowly and holding that breath for a moment and then breathing out. Then again, breathing in slowly and holding before slowly releasing it. Go on with this this breathing technique for a minute or two.

As you breathe, feel your body starting to relax. Feel your body starting to feel heavy, starting to feel comfortable. That heaviness spreads up through your body, from the tips of your toes to the top of your head.

Take yourself back to the top of that beautiful staircase, noticing how safe and inviting it is as you descend … going down deeper … deeper with each step … relaxing more and then more still. You feel heavier and more comfortable than you ever thought possible.

Perhaps you can count those steps down, from twenty to zero, imagining yourself going deeper and deeper still, perhaps curious about what you will find at the bottom of those stairs.

Going down deeper, relaxing … easing … feeling oh so comfortable and so heavy and so relaxed. You do not care if you sleep, you enjoy this relaxation as you go deeper inside yourself.

The deeper you go the more comfortable and more relaxed you become, feeling heavy and detached, relaxed and happy and curious about what you will see at the bottom of your stairs.

The further down you go, the deeper into hypnosis you are. Perhaps you see the door at the bottom of the stairs, allow the door to formulate in your inner vision. Envision the door; the color, the size, the handle, what it is made out of.

Note your feelings. Are you intimidated by what may be behind that door? Are you afraid to walk through the door and face it? Or are you ready to open the door, eager to face whatever is on the other side. You know you have the power to control this world, that you are in the place of the mind-self. You are the master of this domain, and you are in complete control.

You are in complete control.

Open that door and walk through, closing it gently behind you. You will be in a place, having closed the door on any distractions.

Let the shadows rise to reveal that you're not in a room at all. The door has led to an outside realm, a beautiful and fanciful land of bright color and crisp beauty. Hear the birds tweeting, feel the breeze on your face. This is the place of your best self, the best place. Here, all is right and well. It is alive with activity, yet it is tranquil and languid, a place of perfect calm and relaxation.

Every time you go through this door you will discover something different, as you explore the beautiful realms of your subconscious mind. See the amazing misty colors swirling around, walk through a forest and note the fresh woodland smell and the leaves and patterns in the bark of the trees, where the branches intertwine with glimmers of sun shining through. Perhaps you will see a squirrel running up the tree and leaping among the branches before disappearing out of view.

The place is mercurial, changeable, adaptable, flexible. It contorts to your moods, it is the place where mind and body meet. And it is the gateway to all other places, all worlds. Because you are all worlds, and you are the mind-self of this space. From here, wherever you may be, you can open any door to any place or any time, far removed though it may be. You are at the central vortex of all space and time, of all worlds, of all the people you are or have been or could ever be.

Use this power. Use it at your will. It is a power that you and you alone can master for yourself. You can only transport yourself or help others to transport themselves, as I am doing for you now. But you alone hold the key to realizing your own inner vision. Only you can look into your own past. Only you know the pains of your past and the possibilities of your future. Only you can clear those emotional cupboards. Only you can open that door.

So go where only you can go, and do what only you can do. Visit exotic, faraway lands, take an ocean voyage or travel through time and space. Or you could visit a particularly happy memory from your past, or remember an event from your childhood that you had almost forgotten about.

Explore a tropical island out there in the sun and stroll along on the beach or splash in the warm water or relax and bask in the warmth of the summer sun. Go for a hike among the mighty redwoods of the Great Northwest. Visit Stonehenge or London, hear Big Ben ring over the Thames. Compare it to Notre Dame, on the banks of the Seine. Climb Mt. Everest and make it back down; jump from the peak and fly down if you like, or just keep flying and never come down.

This is your special time. Utilize this experience and your creative imagination - to discover the journeys that lie inside you. You have the potential to go wherever you wish, knowing that when it is time to awaken you can do so, feeling calm and refreshed and ready to deal with anything.

Drift off to a place deep inside you, awakening at your regular time, alert and refreshed.

Remember that when your sleep has been interrupted for any reason that does not require your immediate attention, return to your bed or your couch or wherever you may be. Envision that you have been asked to perform a task that you'd rather not do. This could be something like going out in the wind and rain or sweeping leaves from outside your home. It is a task you would like to avoid at all costs, so you pretend to be asleep.

Mimic the actions and inactions of sleep by closing your eyes and breathing deeply and regularly as that warm heavy feeling spreads from the tips of your toes to the top of your head.

Take yourself to the top of that staircase as that heaviness increases and your tired body relaxes and drifts off to its own special place.

You are breathing slowly, rhythmically. As you descend the stairs and the heaviness and relaxation increases, a mist forms in your mind as faint images appear. Those images grow clearer as you embark on a different adventure before drifting back to sleep.

Feel that heaviness come over you, body and mind. Feel your body sink into the sheets, the mattress, the pillow. Feel the comforter wrap around you like your mother's loving embrace. Return to that time of peace in your life, when worry and responsibility were an illusion, where life was but a dream. There can be no distractions in that mindset, nothing will be able to pierce that comforting calm. You find yourself in a peaceful place, a peaceful space. There are no obstacles, nothing standing in the way of your restful repast. You will not toss and turn. You will not be hungry to distraction. Your body is perfectly comfortable, grateful to have this time to do what it needs to do, what it must do to create the best you, the best body for your best mind. This is what your want in body and mind, and what you deserve.

And you have it.

You find that sleep comes easily to you. When you return to bed after being interrupted, your body naturally resumes a comfortable position and you enjoy the rest of your rest.

I'm going to be quiet for a moment as you open that door and step through it to wherever it leads you.

These suggestions are deeply embedded in your subconscious mind. They grow stronger every day. They grow stronger by the day, stronger by the hour, stronger by the minute.

And while your strength increases, so does your power over the things which stood between you and a good night's sleep. The worries, the stresses, none can compete with your newly enlightened will. You will sleep through the night, because your mind will create a world where this happens. That world is your world. That world is you.

You can control your body, and only you can give it what it needs. It needs sleep. It wants sleep. Your mind needs sleep. Your mind wants sleep. And nothing in this world or any other can stop you, can interrupt you. No hunger pangs can get through that comfortable bed. No worries about self-image can violate the snug sanctity of your rest bed. Sleep is like a form of meditation. You focus on one thing, a good night's sleep. You focus on the dark of your closed eyes, the silence of the room around you. The world is sleeping, you too will sleep. Because there is nothing which can stand against your united mind and body, your best and strongest mind-self.

In a moment, I'm going to count you back up to normal conscious awareness. At the count of five you will be wide awake fully alert and refreshed and ready to allow these suggestions to work for you.

One … two … three … coming back slowly. Four … eyelids are fluttering. Five … your eyes are opening, you are wide awake, body mind and body are returning to normal.

Now let's relax and reflect. Where did you go with your special time? How did it feel to be there? What effects were there from your session? When descended into hypnotism, how did it feel? Was the sensation familiar? Did you feel the sensation of heaviness, calmness, ready for sleep? Was your mind peaceful, ready for rest? Do you feel more secure facing a night's sleep? Ae you looking forward to trying them just before bedtime? Are you confident or do you have trepidation? Either is normal, both are positive. They mean you're invested in you efforts, and they mean you have a good chance of success. The great thing is that you can always try again, with this or any of our specialized sessions. They'll become more familiar, easier to manage and more effective. If you made progress with this session, congratulations. If not, congratulations for trying. Even if you had success, try again anyway. That is what this book, what all of our books, are truly all about.

We have taken journeys to the limits of existence and then well beyond that. You now have the power and the experience to travel again, to make such travel a regular part of your life. You will find a richer world within and without. And what you learn will work with your other efforts toward total wellness. Congratulations on breaching that final frontier. You have worked hard and earned the value of the experiences you've had in the realm of the mind-self.

CONCLUSION

Congratulations! You started out this journey with a need, for change and for the knowledge of how to affect that change. Our promise was that if you retained just one significant lesson from this book, it could change your life. All of them could be a revolution for you and for everyone you know. But I'll bet you've picked up much more than that. So it's time for a personal review: Which lessons did you learn the most from? Which was the greater revelation, that cholesterol can be both good and bad, and that each comes from different types of foods? Did you realize how important hormones are to your overall wellness and good health? Did you ever realize you could manipulate your own hormone level and prevent hormonal imbalance? If you did know that, did you realize that some aspects of hormonal function are actually hereditary? Or was it the differences between the different kinds of fats? Was it the fasting? Which type did you try? If both, which worked best? Had you ever heard of autophagy before? How do people react when you explain it to them?

Had you ever practiced yoga before? If you read the book through a first time before applying any of it, are you looking forward to it? Or would meditation be a better place for you to start? At least you're thinking about these things, asking these questions, and that's the key to your ongoing success.

Keep asking these questions, because the nature of this book is to keep you interested and curious, to keep you learning more and teaching more about these things. You may have taken the journey from wanting better health to having it, from ignorance about the benefits and practices of yoga and meditation and exercise. But that journey doesn't really end. From the new perspective of your so-called destination, you can see that life itself is a journey and requires constant progress. As comprehensive as this book is, we acknowledge that it's just the first leg of your journey to wellness.

There will be more scientific breakthrough and discoveries, and your journey calls upon you to be openminded to them. Keep abreast of the new studies, of the cutting edge tech. There are more exercises to learn, more complicated yoga classes, more intense meditative practices.

And when it comes to hypnosis, the sky is genuinely the limit. You've learned to let your mind control your body, but we've given you insight into ways to control your mind in a way you never thought possible. It's just another tool in your wellness toolbox, now it's one you can use.

You can always investigate new ways of thinking and being. You can and you must; you owe it to yourself and to those you love. And this book has shown you the way; it's up to you to make the most of it, to keep going on your journey. But take this book with you, as it has information you will go back to again and again. You may need refreshing as to all the complex facts and concepts. You may need a booster to your confidence. That's okay, everybody needs that from time to time.

But don't let this book be the only one you read. We offer other books on this subject, such as the one which focuses on women. Female bodies have particular needs and complexities which male bodies don't have. There will be some repeated information, but only what is required for complete understanding. There's more to learn, and we're dedicated to helping you through every new stage of your personal development.

Look our catalogue over and see if we don't have books for maladies you may not even know you suffer from. Open your mind and your heart to new avenues, new fields of study, new ways to make yourself a better person and your life a better experience. Helping yourself is a practice which transcends any single aspect of life. And, of course, every facet affects every other facet. These parts of our lives, of ourselves, are interlocked, each touching the other in critical and crucial ways. If this is the one lesson you took away from this book, then that alone is worth the price.

Still, you're now well-informed about dieting, nutrition, exercise, mental expansion, mental and physical unity. And you've seen not just how they work, but *that* they work. Since this is a book to be reread, to be used as a field guide for wellness, you may have read it once through just for a bedrock foundational understanding. You may not have tried any of the exercises yet, or the meditations. And that's excellent. Now you can go back with a sense of familiarity, with fewer questions and greater understanding. The dietary sections of the book aren't meant to be read once and memorized, but to be referred to often. So we encourage you to go back and read it again, to apply the exercises.

Or you might have dived right in and chosen a diet, engaged in some of these programs and exercises. That's great too! Neither approach is wrong if it's right for you. And if you did jump right in, now is the time to step back and reflect. How do you feel? How much better do you feel? How are our cholesterol levels? Did you lose weight? How much?

It's probably something, and that's great. It may not be as much as you'd hoped. But guess what, that's great too! We agreed at the beginning that there were no magic bullets, no overnight miracles. Whatever progress you've made is proof positive that these exercises, diets, and other applications work. The more they are implemented, the more they will continue to work. Let your progress be your guide. Keep it up! You should have a new sense of empowerment and capability. You should have more energy and endurance to accomplish even more. Fast longer, exercise harder, be more mindful and more deliberate.

But remember or caveats: Good change is gradual change. Always transition into and out of any dietary or exercise application in the macro and the micro. Always consult a physician before starting a new dietary and/or exercise protocol. Keep in touch with your doctor too, to note any changes and make sure no damage is being done. Never overstress your body and mind; stress is good for your body, as it instigates change. Too much stress is harmful, as it can damage muscle, bone, and organ function. Remember that you're on a journey, and every so-called *destination* is just a waystation on the way to something bigger, someone better.

Keep up your journey, wherever it takes you. Every journey will be unique to the person taking it. Every discovery will reveal a new challenge, every destination points out the next road to travel. Along the way, you'll travel with more strength, more energy, more people following you. At the end, you'll find that idealized life and self you're working toward. Though chances are, once you've achieved that you'll only want to move forward still, improving things time and again. There's always room for improvement; and, as always, we'll be there with you every step of the way.

So let's keep going!

RESOURCES

https://getkion.com/blogs/all/intermittent-fasting-weight-loss

https://getkion.com/blogs/all/how-to-fast

https://getkion.com/blogs/all/breaking-a-fast-mindfully

https://intermittentdieter.com/best-foods-to-break-a-fast/

https://www.healthline.com/health/autophagy

https://www.medicalnewstoday.com/articles/autophagy#health-effects

https://www.whitneyerd.com/2020/01/the-truth-about-autophagy.html

https://paleoleap.com/long-fasts/

https://www.healthline.com/nutrition/6-ways-to-do-intermittent-fasting

https://www.jagranjosh.com/general-knowledge/list-of-important-hormones-and-their-functions-1516176713-1

https://www.hormone.org/your-health-and-hormones/glands-and-hormones-a-to-z

https://www.healthline.com/health/hormonal-imbalance#hair-loss

https://www.healthline.com/health/hormonal-imbalance#other-complications

https://www.ncbi.nlm.nih.gov/pmc/articles/PMC4445642/

https://www.arbor-health.com/blog/estrogen-dominance

https://www.uclahealth.org/endocrine-center/genetic-syndromes

https://health.clevelandclinic.org/are-you-planning-a-cleanse-or-detox-read-this-first/

https://www.healthline.com/nutrition/how-to-detox-your-body#The-Bottom-Line

https://skinkraft.com/blogs/articles/toxic-chemicals-in-cosmetics

https://thefoxandshe.com/skincare-ingredients-to-avoid/

https://experiencelife.lifetime.life/article/8-hidden-toxins-whats-lurking-in-your-cleaning-products/

https://www.lovense.com/bdsm-blog/enema-solutions

https://draxe.com/health/coffee-enema/

https://www.everydayhealth.com/diet-and-nutrition/diet/detox-cleanses-most-popular-types-what-know/

https://www.byrdie.com/best-juice-cleanses-4800007

https://www.cookinglight.com/eating-smart/clean-eating/3-cleanses-you-should-never-do-and-3-worth-trying

https://www.gaiam.com/blogs/discover/10-ways-to-detoxify-your-body

https://www.healthline.com/health/type-2-diabetes-ketogenic-diet

https://intermittentdieter.com/best-foods-to-break-a-fast/

https://www.mayoclinic.org/healthy-lifestyle/nutrition-and-healthy-eating/in-depth/paleo-diet/art-20111182

https://www.medicalnewstoday.com/articles/324405

https://www.webmd.com/diet/atkins-diet-what-you-can-eat#3

https://www.atkins.com/how-it-works/library/articles/7-day-keto-meal-plan

https://www.mayoclinic.org/diseases-conditions/diabetes/in-depth/diabetes-diet/art-20044295

https://www.marksdailyapple.com/how-to-exercise-while-fasting/

https://www.menshealth.com/fitness/a30300614/intermittent-fasting-working-out/

https://www.webmd.com/diet/a-z/hormone-diet

https://www.eatingwell.com/article/7805452/hormone-balancing-foods-how-diet-can-help/

https://www.health.harvard.edu/staying-healthy/the-truth-about-fats-bad-and-good

https://www.heart.org/en/healthy-living/healthy-eating/eat-smart/fats/dietary-fats

https://health.clevelandclinic.org/where-does-body-fat-go-when-you-lose-weight/

https://www.prevention.com/fitness/g20459708/best-workouts-to-target-belly-fat/

https://www.keckmedicine.org/what-is-the-difference-between-good-and-bad-cholesterol/

https://yogasynergy.com/article-on-fasting-and-yoga-by-john-mcwhorter/

https://dailycup.yoga/2019/11/10/why-you-should-consider-fasting-4-tips-to-prepare-for-your-first-fast/

https://www.chandriniyoga.com/blog/2018/4/29/the-practice-of-yoga-while-fasting

https://www.juruyoga.com/the-practice-of-yoga-while-fasting/

https://www.yogadownload.com/Utilities/ProgramDisplay/tabid/359/prodid/13004#.YH0Alz9lBPY

https://glennfay.medium.com/intermittent-fasting-and-meditation-remedies-for-weight-management-acdbf53ba76c

https://medium.com/the-ascent/meditation-intermittent-fasting-for-the-mind-7ab6a98cdb23

https://ourworldindata.org/obesity#what-are-the-drivers-of-obesity

https://www.ncbi.nlm.nih.gov/pmc/articles/PMC6347410/

https://www.healthline.com/nutrition/top-13-evidence-based-health-benefits-of-coffee#TOC_TITLE_HDR_5

https://courses.lumenlearning.com/introchem/chapter/hydrogenation/

https://booksy.com/blog/us/what-is-holistic-medicine-and-why-should-i-care/

https://www.nhs.uk/live-well/exercise/exercise-health-benefits/

https://www.hypno-fasting.com/faq

https://hypnotc.com/hypnotherapy-fasting-weight-loss/

https://www.verywellmind.com/best-hypnosis-apps-4800547

https://www.hypnotherapy-london.info/the-history-of-hypnosis/

https://www.spaceotechnologies.com/best-intermittent-fasting-apps/

https://www.tomsguide.com/best-picks/best-workout-apps

https://www.verywellfit.com/best-yoga-apps-4176689

https://www.nhs.uk/live-well/exercise/exercise-health-benefits/

https://www.hypnoticworld.com/hypnosis-scripts/

https://www.mayoclinic.org/healthy-lifestyle/nutrition-and-healthy-eating/in-depth/vegetarian-diet/art-20046446

https://www.tasteofhome.com/collection/vegetarian-meal-plan/

Lightning Source UK Ltd.
Milton Keynes UK
UKHW020634210521
384122UK00013B/929